Historic Hospitals of Long Beach

GERRIE SCHIPSKE, R.N.P., J.D.

AMERICA THROUGH TIME®
ADDING COLOR TO AMERICAN HISTORY

Front cover photo: The Naval Hospital, Long Beach, was commissioned in December 1942 and opened in 1943 to treat personnel wounded in the Pacific Theater. It closed in 1950 and then became the Veteran's Administration Hospital. (*US Naval Medicine*)

Back cover photo: The construction crew that built the Community Hospital was supervised by Herbert Murphy. Forty years later, Murphy joined the Community Hospital Association Board of Directors. (*CHLBF*)

America Through Time is an imprint of Fonthill Media LLC
www.through-time.com
office@through-time.com

Published by Arcadia Publishing by arrangement with Fonthill Media LLC
For all general information, please contact Arcadia Publishing:
Telephone: 843-853-2070
Fax: 843-853-0044
E-mail: sales@arcadiapublishing.com
For customer service and orders:
Toll-Free 1-888-313-2665

www.arcadiapublishing.com

First published 2019

ISBN 978-1-63499-094-3

Typeset in 10pt on 13pt Sabon
Printed and bound in England

Preface

Writing this book seemed to be the next logical step in my quest to chronicle my affection for the place where I was born, work and raise a family. While researching it, I found many connections in my life with the history of these hospitals: In 1950, I was one of the "last babies" delivered at the U.S. Naval Hospital on 7th Street (now the VA); I did a portion of my nursing training at Memorial Medical Center (where my son was later born) and managed "patient relations" at St. Mary Medical Center (where my youngest daughter was born); I served on the City of Long Beach Board of Health for over nine years; served as a trustee for the Long Beach Community College District which operates one of the oldest nursing programs in the area; as a City Council member, I voted to allow Memorial Medical Center to operate Community Hospital to save the hospital from closing; and today, I teach healthcare administration at California State University at Long Beach, on the same land where the Tongva, the first "healers" of Long Beach, lived.

Discovering the history of the Long Beach hospitals that provide care and treatment for the people who lived here gave me a new appreciation of the generous spirit of this city. Few cities in the United States stepped up and built a "community hospital" to serve its residents. Even fewer cities set public health as one of its first priorities when incorporating. Because of the philanthropy of Adelaide Tichenor in the 1920s, children have been able to receive care through the Tichenor Orthopedic Clinic. The gift of city land made it possible for the U.S. Navy to operate hospitals to care for the sick and wounded during times of war and peace.

As this book is published, the City of Long Beach once again struggles with the possible closure of Long Beach Community Hospital. Faced with the staggering costs of retrofitting several of its buildings to withstand earthquakes, Memorial Medical Center chose to no longer operate the facility in 2018.

Long Beach's history is proof that it is a city that is strong and caring. No doubt, it will continue to find a way to support its community hospital.

ACKNOWLEDGMENTS

The words and photographs in this book would not have been possible without the encouragement of Matthew Faulkner, Executive Director, Community Hospital Long Beach Foundation, the persistence of Matthew Rodriguez from Fonthill, the wonderful archives and staff of the Historical Society of Long Beach and Long Beach Public Library and the understanding of my family.

Contents

INTRODUCTION

Residents of Long Beach, like most Americans in the early twentieth century, gave birth, treated illness and even underwent surgery, at home. Hospitals were considered places for the poor and the severely infirm or places to quarantine contagious disease.

This seaside resort advertised its temperate climate and became home for numerous sanitariums offering rest, "light therapy," mineral baths and "milk cures." As physicians became more professional, they pushed for a regular hospital. It would take until 1906 for the Long Beach Hospital to open. A year later, Seaside Hospital offered twelve patient rooms.

Long Beach soon became the "fastest growing city" by luring visitors with the Pine Avenue Pier, the Walk of a Thousand Lights and the Pacific Railroad. Thousands came; many stayed. The discovery of oil in 1921 brought considerable wealth and workers to the city.

The Catholic population grew, and a local parish priest invited the Sisters of Charity of the Incarnate Word to come from Texas and repurpose the Long Beach Sanitarium into St. Mary's Hospital. They did in 1923.

Oilman and anti-saloon advocate, Fillmore Condit, came to Long Beach, after dropping out of running for governor of New Jersey. Almost immediately, Condit was elected to the Long Beach City Council and became the strongest "champion" for a "community hospital." With substantial financial support from the City of Long Beach and community groups, including the KKK, Long Beach Community Hospital opened in 1924 with seventy beds.

Former public health officer, Dr. Harriman Jones, opened a private practice on Daisy Avenue and then moved to land owned by Park Nursery on Broadway and Junipero where he established the Harriman Jones Clinic and Hospital in 1930.

Accidents, epidemics and other tragedies sent many to the local hospitals. When the 1933 earthquake hit, it devastated most of Long Beach schools as well as Seaside and St. Mary's. Only Community withstood the shaking.

The Navy ported at Long Beach and military airplanes were manufactured at Douglas Aircraft Plant, and once again, the population soared. A Ferry Command Station Hospital and a U.S. Naval Hospital were opened and after the war became the Long Beach General Hospital and Veterans Administration Hospital. A second Naval hospital opened in 1972 and closed twenty years later.

Despite opposition from the medical profession, osteopaths flourished in Long Beach from its start and opened several hospitals and maternity clinics.

Seaside became Seaside Memorial Hospital and in 1960 opened "the first space age hospital" in the middle of the city. Today, Memorial Medical Center of Long Beach includes Miller Children's Hospital and is the largest hospital in the city. St. Mary's Hospital continued to expand and in 1975 became St. Mary Medical Center.

"The people's hospital"—Community Hospital of Long Beach—expanded and survived most of the financial challenges it faced. In 2018, its operator, Memorial Medical Center, announced that it would not be able to meet the seismic retrofit requirements imposed by the State and terminated its lease with the City of Long Beach. The future of Community Hospital is uncertain at the time of this publication.

1

The History of Places of Healing

O, my ancestor, O, my ancestor, listen to my heart, O' my ancestor, here is my heart.
From Tongva honor song

Long before there were hospitals in Long Beach, California, there were "natural" healers. The Tongva Native Americans inhabited the southern Los Angeles basin and relied heavily upon medicinal plants for their healing practices. Tongva means "people of the earth." The Tongva were renamed San Gabriel Mission Indians or Gabrielinos-Tongva after the Mission San Gabriel Arcangel, where they were forced to work the land and tend cattle and sheep after the Spanish settled the area.

A Tongva sacred place lies in the eastern portion of Long Beach—on the grounds of Rancho Los Alamitos and California State University at Long Beach. Known as Puvunga (also called Pubuna), the site is the birthplace of the Tongva lawgiver and god, Chengiichngech. Daily personal bathing and cleaning of *kiis* (huts) were part of his teaching.

Pitzer College in Claremont, California, features a "Tongva Native Garden" that includes twenty-three plants and trees identified as having medicinal properties. Mark Acuna, a Tongva ethno-botanist, catalogued plants used by the Tongva for medicinal use: white and black sage, sagebrush, buckwheat, chamise, yucca, agave, white alder, manzanita, sycamore, mule fat, gooseberry, coastal oak, lilac, deer grass and willow.

Unfortunately, European diseases took their toll and many natives and new settlers died. Early non-native settlers of Long Beach in the 1880s relied upon the women in their families during times of illness or childbirth. Women provided home remedies and only on rare occasions was a local physician summoned to the home.

Physicians were in short supply and those who practiced only had a year of training. Physicians knew limited procedures for helping the sick and relied upon bloodletting, blistering, giving arsenic and mercury, enemas and purges. While antibiotics would not be discovered until the turn of the twentieth century, the discovery of anesthesia meant that more surgery could be performed, which increased the demand for hospitals. For many years, hospitals continued to be places only for the poor and were either public or run by Catholic nuns.

Medicine took a giant leap because of the Civil War. Most of the 55,000 physicians in the U.S. had little training in handling battlefield trauma or mass communicable disease.

More than 15,000 physicians served in the Union and Confederate armies. To deal with the mass casualties and disparities in training, the military imposed standardized protocols for treatment and removed from use the deadly compounds containing mercury, calomel and antimony.

The work of the volunteer U.S. Sanitary Commission during the Civil War improved the health and sanitary conditions of the military camps and field hospitals. The Commission was headed by men, but most of the volunteer work was conducted by women.

At the end of the war, the railroads owned millions of acres of land given to them by the government. The railroads were eager to sell the land and at the same time to stop the flow of immigrants from China. Even though the railroads had exploited Chinese labor to build the railroads across the country, they wanted them out of California.

The California Immigrant Union (CIU) was established to market the railroad land and to attract white, Christian families from Europe and the east coast of the U.S. Its pamphlet explained:

> We need population—not of races inferior in natural traits, pagan in religion, ignorant of free institutions and incapable of sharing in them without putting the very existence of those institutions in peril—but we need immigrants of kindred races who will constitute a congenial element and locate themselves and their families permanently upon the soil; who can be admitted to an equal share in our political privileges, and respond to all the obligations imposed upon citizens under a republican government.

As physicians received more formalized training, they began recognizing the connection between hand washing and prevention of disease. Public health became important in the promotion of sanitation, sewers, vaccination and dealing with communicable diseases.

Physicians organized through medical associations. They became known as professionals and were accorded higher stature in their communities. The medical profession was challenged by "osteopathic physicians." Osteopaths focused their practice on the realignment of "misplaced bones" or "osteopathic lesions," along the spinal column. It was thought that these lesions interfered with nerves, including those that regulated an adequate blood supply. This theory was detailed in the 1901 publication of *Osteopathic Physician* titled "Most Diseases Are of Spinal Origin."

Patients knew little about the difference between an M.D. and a D.O. In 1902, the "Resident and Classified Directory of Greater Long Beach" listed thirty-four physicians and five osteopathic physicians. By 1907, forty-two physicians and thirteen osteopathic physicians were on the list.

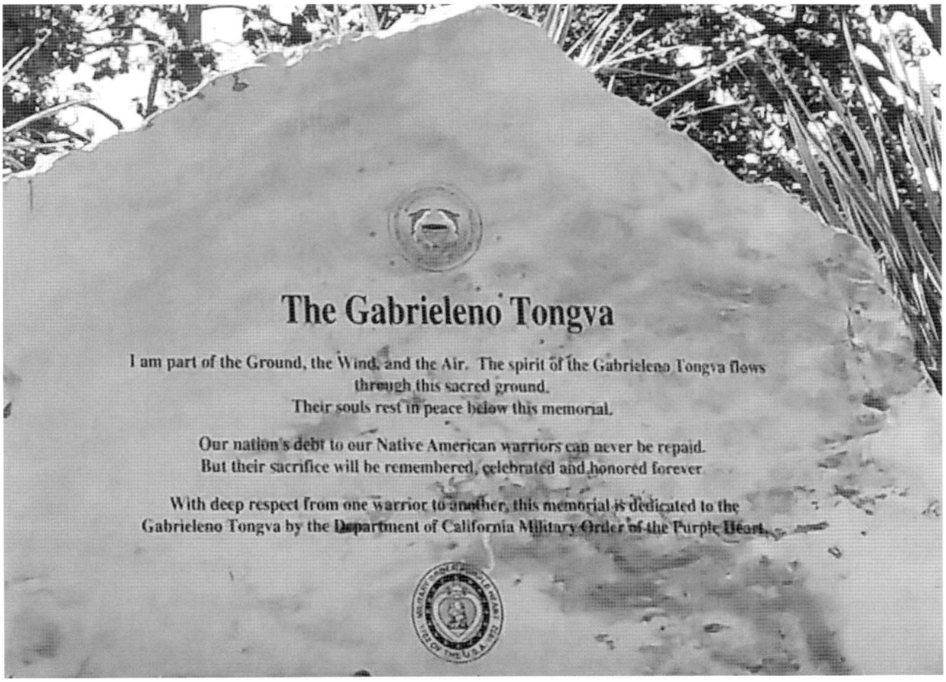
The Gabrieleno Tongva
I am part of the Ground, the Wind, and the Air. The spirit of the Gabrieleno Tongva flows through this sacred ground.
Their souls rest in peace below this memorial.
Our nation's debt to our Native American warriors can never be repaid.
But their sacrifice will be remembered, celebrated and honored forever.
With deep respect from one warrior to another, this memorial is dedicated to the Gabrieleno Tongva by the Department of California Military Order of the Purple Heart.

The Tongva are celebrated on two markers on the grounds of the Veterans Administration Medical Center in east Long Beach. This area is part of the Rancho Los Alamitos on which the sacred Puvunga was located.

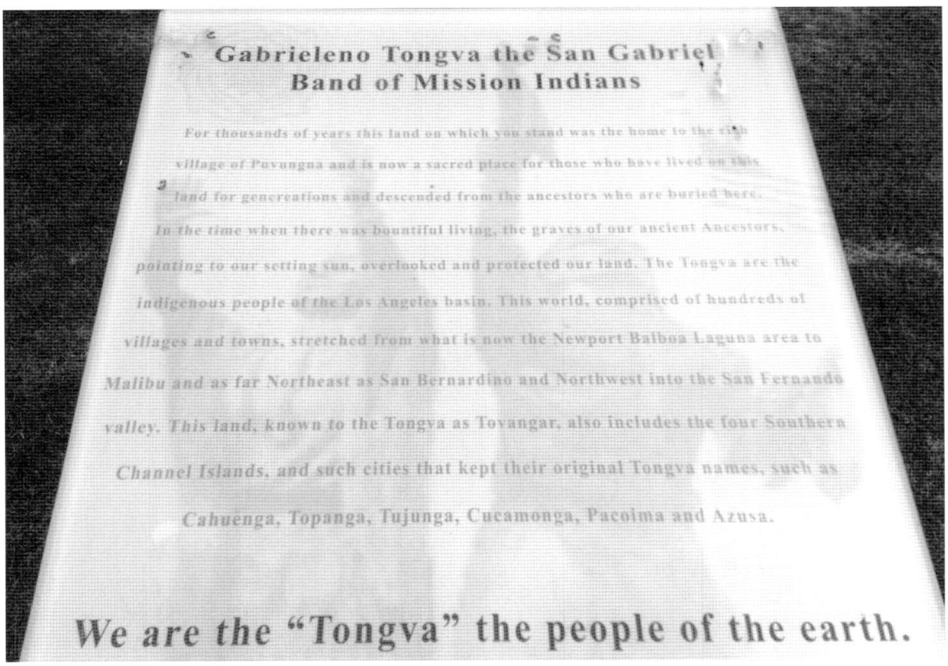

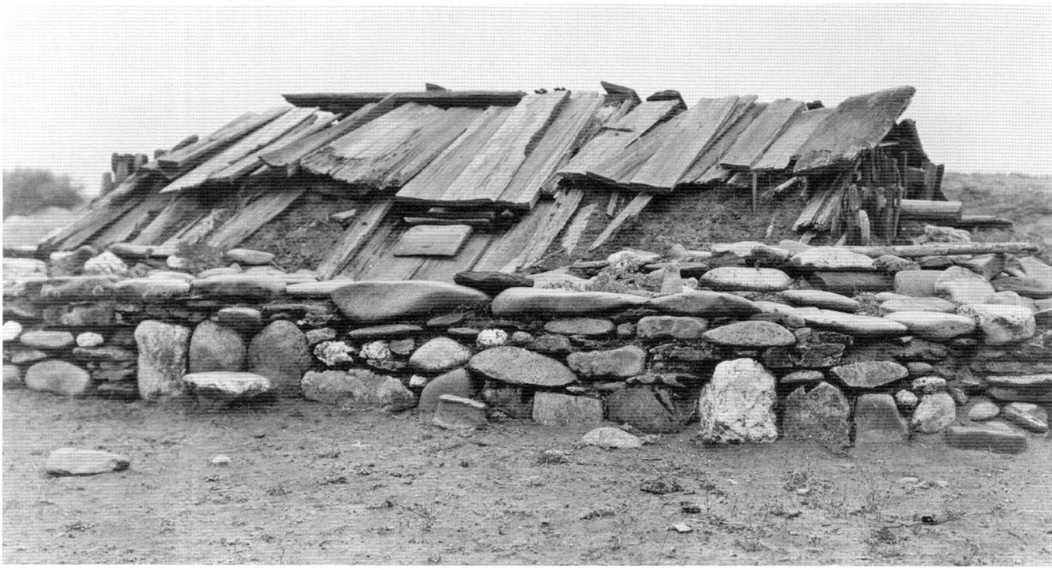

The abundant willow tree contains "salicin" which is an ingredient of aspirin that provides pain and fever relief. The wood of the willow was also utilized to construct "sweat houses" that enabled the ill to purify and rid themselves of illness. (*LOC*)

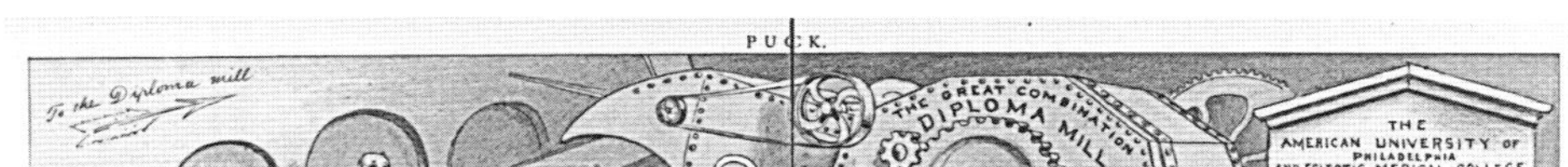

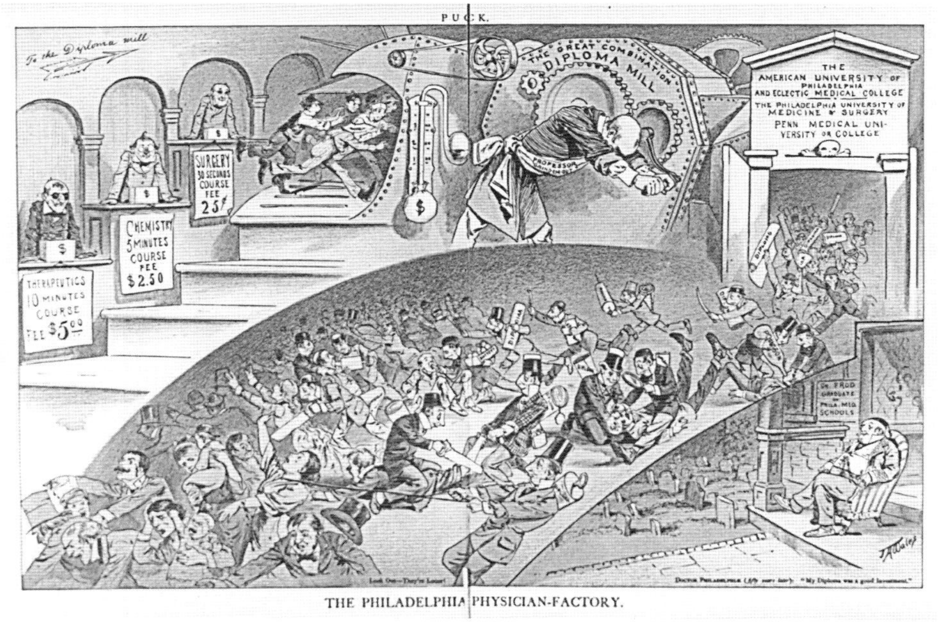

In early Long Beach, there were few physicians, and most were poorly trained because of the lack of standards. Many in the profession complained that medical schools were nothing more than "physician factories" or "diploma mills" as illustrated in this 1890s drawing from *Puck* magazine. (*LOC*)

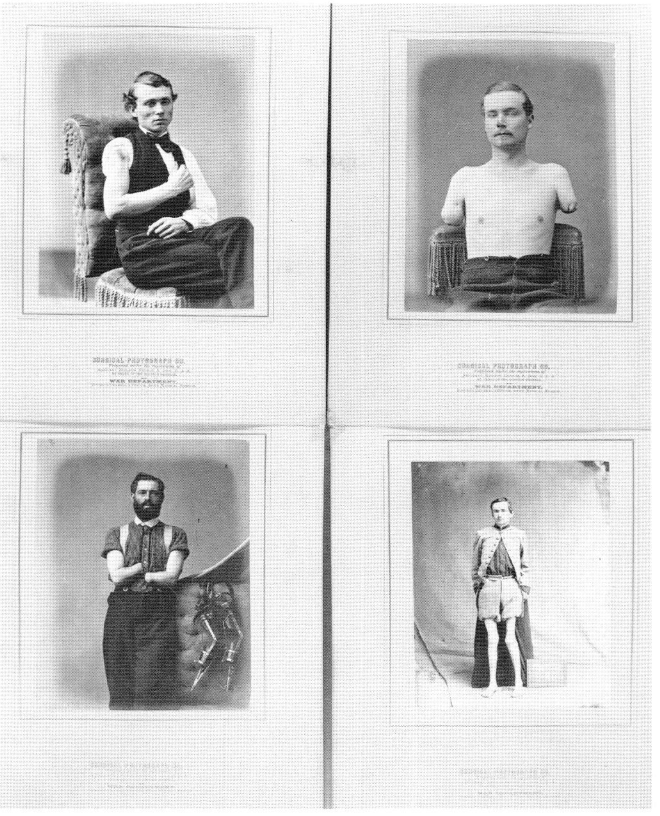

Of the estimated 700,000 deaths during the Civil War, more than 400,000 were caused by communicable disease, dysentery or infected wounds. Guns and cannons took their toll, requiring surgeons to perform amputations without anesthesia or antibiotic. The U.S. War Department and U.S. Surgeon General documented the types of amputations in this Library of Congress photograph.

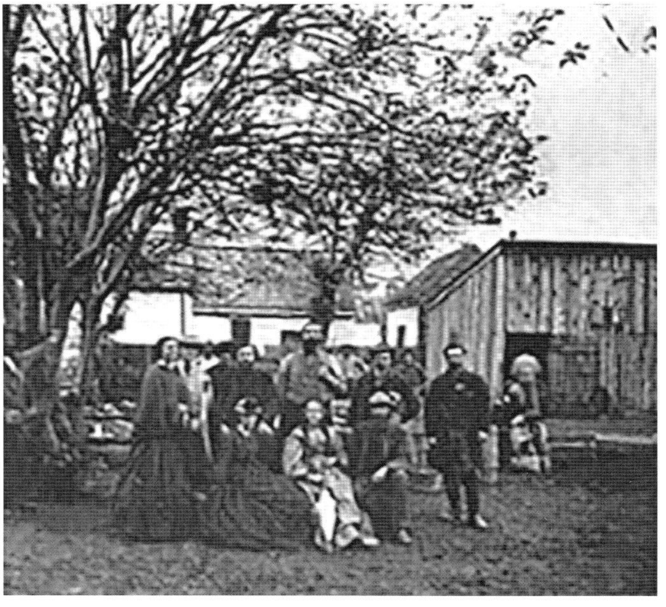

In 1861, the United States Sanitary Commission (USSC) was formed by volunteers to inspect the conditions in the military camps and field hospitals. Their efforts made significant changes in hospital care. The organization was run by men, but most of the volunteer work was done by women who nursed the sick and wounded. This photograph shows nurses and officers at a field hospital in Fredericksburg, Virginia. (*LOC*)

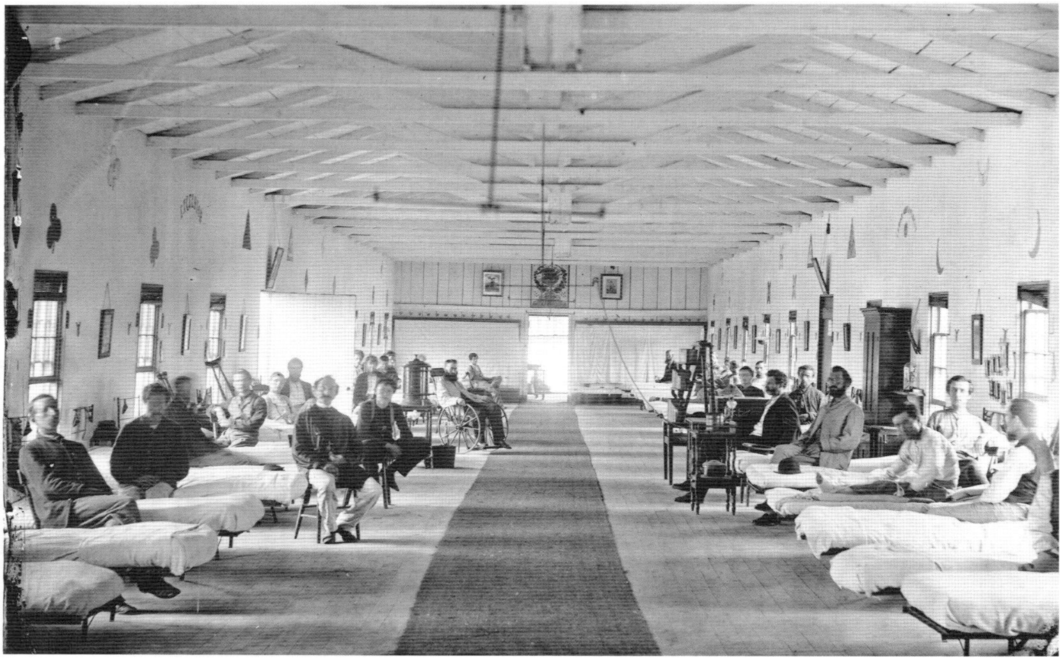

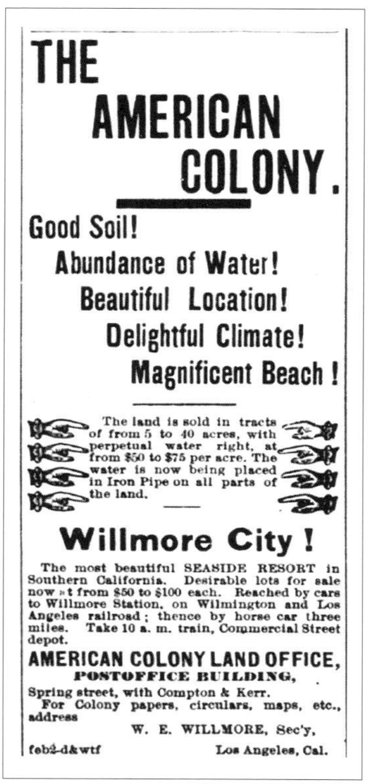

Above: The women of the USSC held "Sanitary Fairs" across the Union states to raise more than $4.9 million in cash and $15 million in supplies. Medical advice was provided by volunteer physicians who wrote and illustrated pamphlets on sanitation and hygiene which could be read by military surgeons. The work done by women in the Civil War significantly changed women's roles in medicine. By the end of the war, the Army employed more 15,000 women as nurses. (*LOC*)

Left: It took until the late 1800s for physicians to understand the connection between hand-washing and preventing infection. The "germ theory" replaced the "bad air theory." People, particularly on the East Coast, were encouraged to go out west to seaside resorts that offered abundant sunshine and fresh air. The American Colony (which became Long Beach) was marketed as the perfect, healthy setting.

2

Early Healthcare in Long Beach

> Long Beach has no rival on the Pacific coast line, with a climate that is always delightful and especially suited for the reinvigoration of invalids, and that acts as a stimulus to those in full health ...
>
> *Los Angeles Herald*, June 19, 1892

The Spanish took the land from the Tongva and other native people and gave it to their friends. The land that includes what is today Long Beach was originally known as Ranchos Los Alamitos and Los Cerritos.

Jotham Bixby, an early non-native settler of the area, was a founding member of the California Immigrant Union (CIU) board. In 1879, he began selling and leasing areas of his Rancho Los Cerritos. Thousands of families responded to the CIU marketing and took advantage of the low fares that were used to entice them to relocate. CIU Manager, William Willmore, leased land from Jotham Bixby and began the American Colony which became "Willmore City." In 1884, after failing to develop the colony, Willmore moved to Texas and the land was purchased by real estate developers and businessmen. Belle Lowe, the wife of a prominent merchant, suggested the area be named "long beach" because of the 8-mile stretch of sand that fronted the town.

Several former Civil War physicians relocated to Long Beach. Among them were Dr. Harry Z. Fretz Gill, who served as surgeon-in-chief of the First Division of the 20th Army Corps.

California established a Board of Health in 1870 to make sanitary investigations and find the sources of diseases. It also dealt with sewage, sanitation, ventilation, interment of the dead and public vaccination.

One of the first actions taken by the newly incorporated City of Long Beach in 1897 was the formation of a "Board of Public Health." Only three cities in California operate their own health department: Long Beach, Berkeley and Pasadena. The City Trustees appointed former Civil War first assistant surgeon, William L. Cuthbert, as its first Public Health Officer in 1898. The Cuthbert's were a close-knit family that came from Belle Plaine, Kansas. Dr. Cuthbert and his entire family played in the "Cuthbert Family Band" and provided concerts in the city's parks and at many church events.

In 1875, Dr. John Kellogg served as the medical director of a sanitorium in Battle Creek, Michigan, and began promoting facilities where patients could "learn to stay well." Consequently, he changed the name "sanitorium" to "sanitarium" to emphasize that the facility was a sanitary, clean place. The Kellogg Sanitarium movement had its basis in Seventh Day Adventist beliefs and promoted the "comforts of home and hotel." Baths of "every description" were provided as well as treatments with electricity and "careful regulation of diet."

Sanitariums became popular with the promotion of the theory that "bad air" or "miasma" caused disease. This theory prompted numerous "scientific" and newspaper articles touting the need for "sunshine and clean air"—both of which were in great quantities in the seaside resort of Long Beach.

Russian born Dr. Michael A. Schutz opened The Long Beach Sanitarium and Hotel Riviera at 333 W. Broadway (corner of Broadway and Chestnut) in 1901. Schutz was a graduate of the University of Southern California. The sanitarium offered treatment for "chronic, nervous and female diseases." It also provided nursing training. Schutz was known for his avid promotion of Long Beach as a tourist destination. He was also involved in creating a "spiritualist temple" at 415 Linden Avenue. Schutz closed his sanitarium in 1918 and moved to Elsinore, California.

In 1905, Dr. W. L. Woodruff opened the "Woodruff Sanatorium" on Pacific Avenue facing the ocean and a park. He practiced homeopathic medicine and offered treatment with electric lights and sunlight. Woodruff adamantly opposed requiring school children to be vaccinated. Several members of the Long Beach Board of Education agreed with him and declared that children did not have to have shots before attending school. Woodruff's fight went statewide and in 1907 the state and local public health officials ordered the vaccination of children. He died in 1910 from a ruptured lung caused by an obese patient falling on him.

As the tourist and resident population of the city swelled, several other sanitariums opened. The Porter Milk Diet Sanitarium opened in 1907 at 737 Sunrise Boulevard. Dr. Charles Porter was the author of the book *Milk Diet as a Remedy for Chronic Disease*, which promoted a diet of three weeks of only raw milk. Porter closed the sanitarium in 1924, complaining that not enough people believed such a simple thing as milk could cure disease.

For several years, Long Beach city trustees and local businessmen discussed establishing a regular hospital. In 1906, the Long Beach Hospital was completed as designed by local architect Harry F. Starbuck. Starbuck also designed the Schutz Sanitarium. Long Beach Hospital's location on 10th Street and Linden Avenue provided an unblocked view of the ocean.

By 1910, the Long Beach Hospital closed and was turned into a sanitarium by W. Ray Simpson. According to several newspaper accounts, the closure of the hospital was caused by "mismanagement and scandals creeping in." Simpson and his wife were later found liable by the California Supreme Court for exerting undue influence on a patient. They coerced her to sign over her entire estate to remain at the sanitarium. Simpson sold the facility to Dr. Truman Boyd in 1921. It remained a sanitarium until it was purchased in 1923 by the Sisters of Charity of the Incarnate Word, who established St. Mary's Hospital.

Right: Once the railroads finished exploiting immigrant Chinese labor to complete the rail system, they mounted efforts to actively remove them. The railroads formed the California Immigrant Union to market the vast acreage and to recruit "white, Christians" from Europe and the East Coast of the U.S. (*CL*)

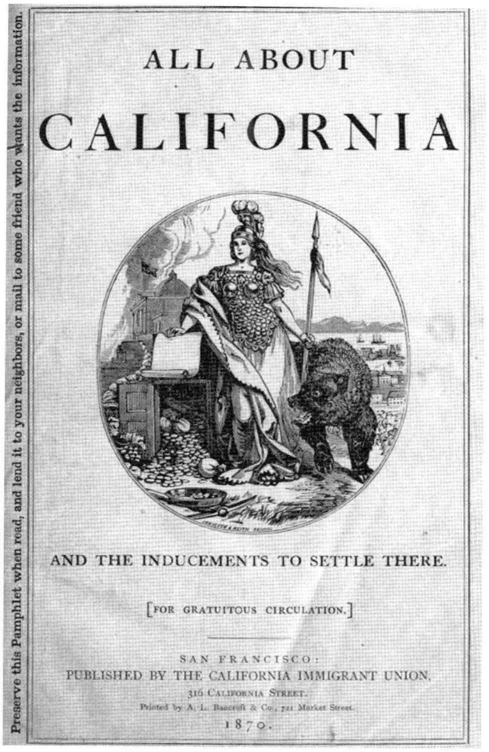

Preserve this Pamphlet when read, and lend it to your neighbors, or mail to some friend who wants the information.

ALL ABOUT

CALIFORNIA

AND THE INDUCEMENTS TO SETTLE THERE.

[FOR GRATUITOUS CIRCULATION.]

SAN FRANCISCO:
PUBLISHED BY THE CALIFORNIA IMMIGRANT UNION,
316 CALIFORNIA STREET.
Printed by A. L. Bancroft & Co., 721 Market Street.
1870.

Below: The railroads often lowered fares to entice passengers to make the journey to view land for sale by including the price of a ticket in the first payment made on the land purchased by the passenger. The area that was to become Long Beach was part of the Spanish land grants: Rancho Los Alamitos and Rancho Los Cerritos. The main railroad station in Long Beach is pictured.

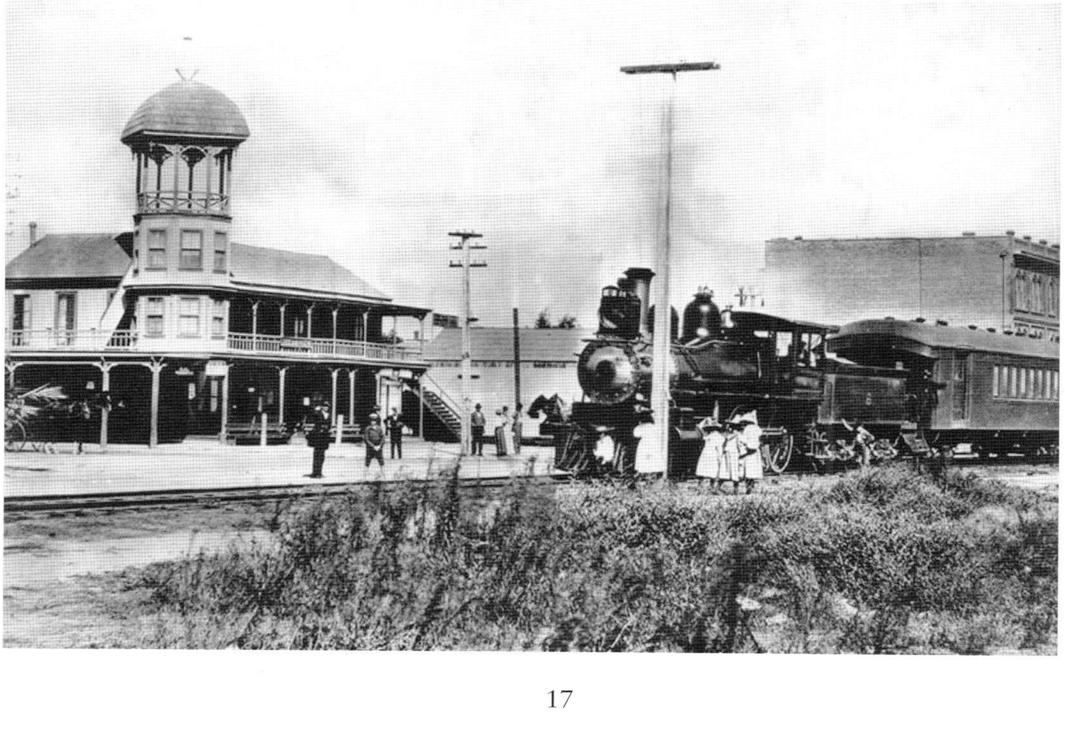

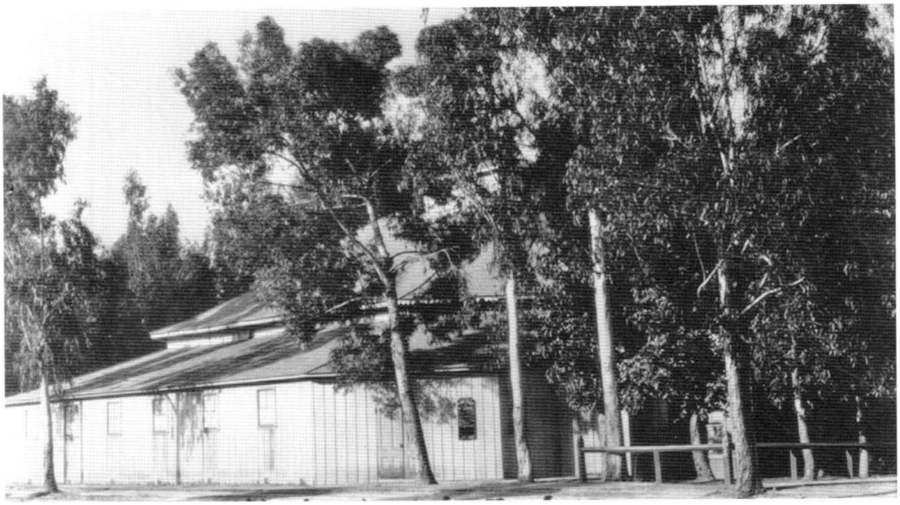

Part of William E. Willmore's plan was to attract members of the Methodist Church to the American Colony in hopes they would purchase land. Willmore included acreage for the Methodist Tabernacle (pictured), where Methodists held their summer "Chautauqua" camps.

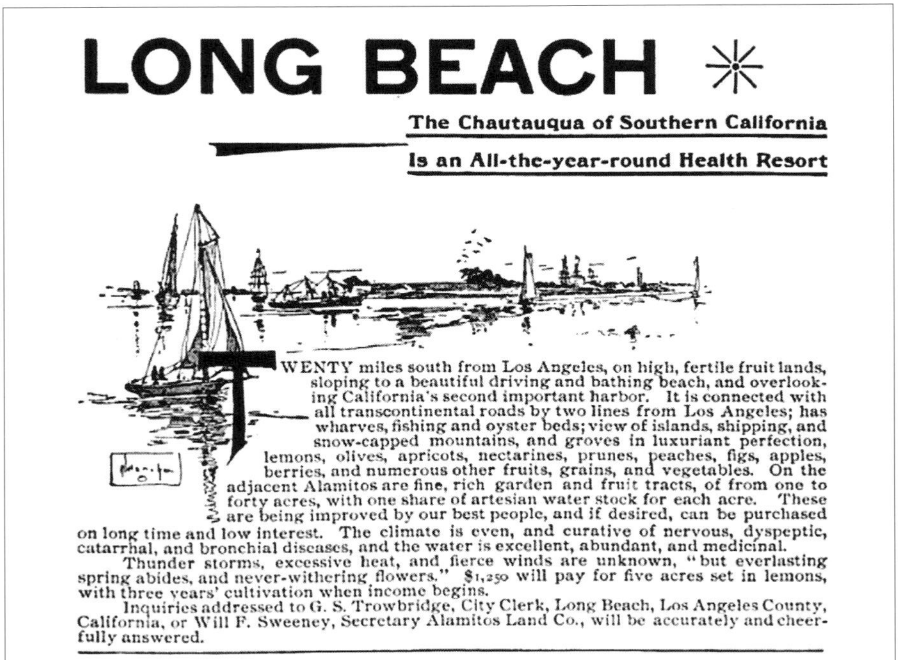

Long Beach became popular with Methodists as "an all-the-year-round health resort." Pamphlets (pictured) for the "Chautauqua of Southern California" described Long Beach as being located "twenty miles from Los Angeles on high, fertile fruit land, sloping to a beautiful driving and bathing beach ... " The city was also known as the "saloon-less seaside resort" because of local laws against alcohol within city limits.

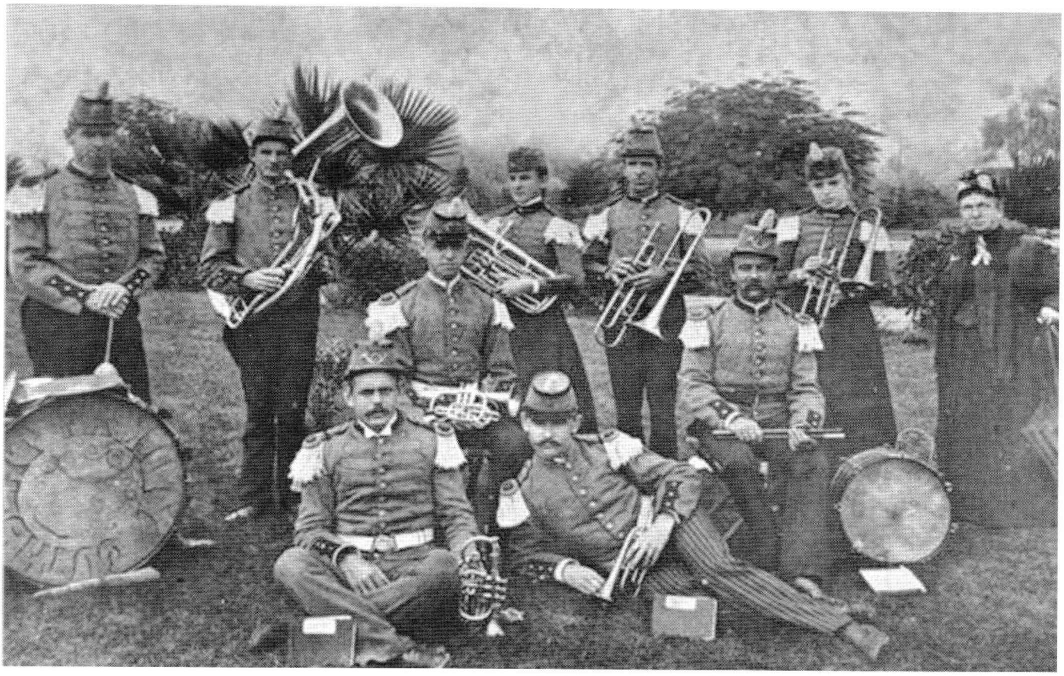

Above: In 1897, Long Beach established its Board of Health and in 1898, appointed Dr. William L. Cuthbert, a former Civil War first assistant surgeon, the city's first public health officer. Cuthbert and his family moved from Belle Plaine, Kansas, to join relatives in Long Beach. In addition to serving as the city's public health officer, Cuthbert formed a family band in 1901 and performed with his wife, sons and daughters in local parks and churches. Cuthbert played both horn and drum.

Right: The medical profession continued to struggle with types of care and treatment to provide. The Seventh Day Adventists developed a "healthy nutrition" approach to treating illness focusing on hygiene, temperance, vegetarianism and natural remedies. In Battle Creek, Michigan, a young doctor, John Kellogg, served as superintendent of the Western Reform Health Institute. Kellogg developed peanut butter, granola and corn flakes to aid digestion. In 1911, the Western Reform Health Institute became "Battle Creek Sanitarium." Kellogg franchised "Battle Creek Sanitariums" across the U.S.

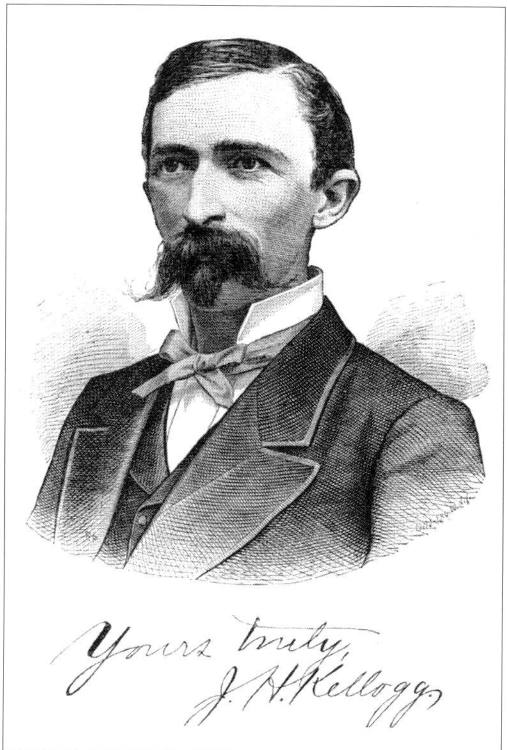

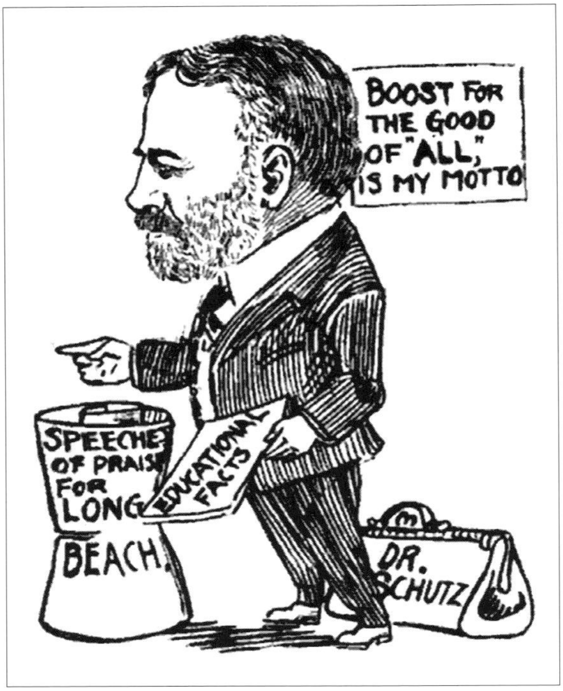

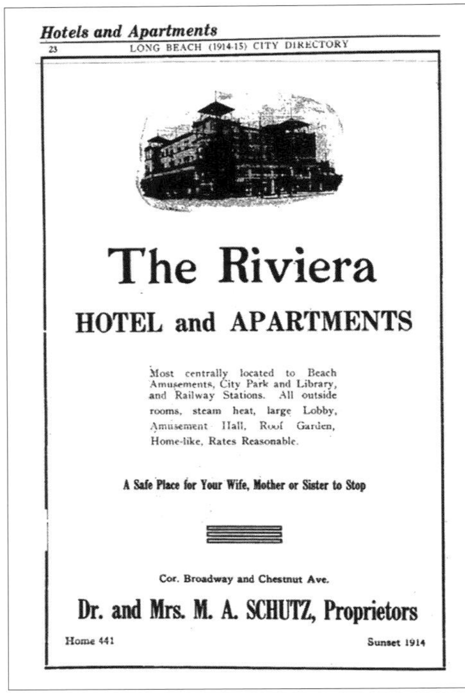

Above left and right: In 1901, Long Beach physician and promoter, Dr. Michael A. Schutz, formed the Long Beach Hotel and Sanitarium Company and opened a sanitarium and Hotel Riviera at Broadway and Chestnut Avenue. Schutz had been encouraged by a friend to move to Long Beach because of the tourists that came each summer for the Methodist camp. His caricature was featured in a 1912 *Out West* magazine as one of Long Beach's most prominent. The once elegant Hotel and Sanitarium at 333 W. Broadway was prominently advertised the in the city directory.

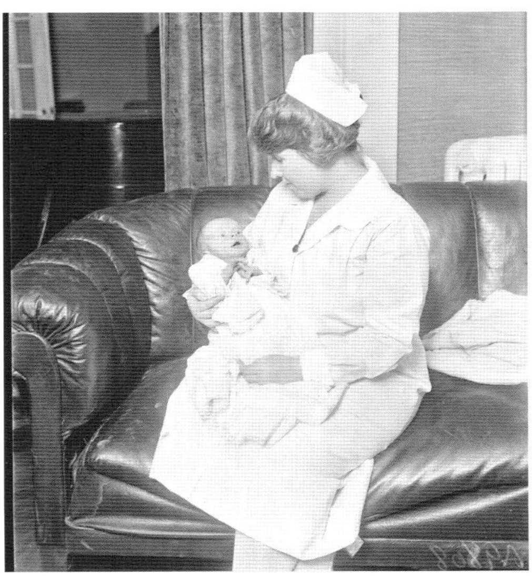

The Schutz Sanitarium also trained nurses. In the early 1900s nursing was still considered to be a "calling" and not a profession. Nursing was thought to be part of a woman's nature. Training was more of an apprenticeship at which young women did most of the care of a patient and the cleaning the facility. Experienced nurses sought private duty assignments with families as shown in this early-1900s photograph. Nurses either cared for patients in the patient's home or accompanied them when they were hospitalized. The more experienced nurses became "matrons" or administrators and were responsible for supervising the staff and scheduling procedures. (*LOC*)

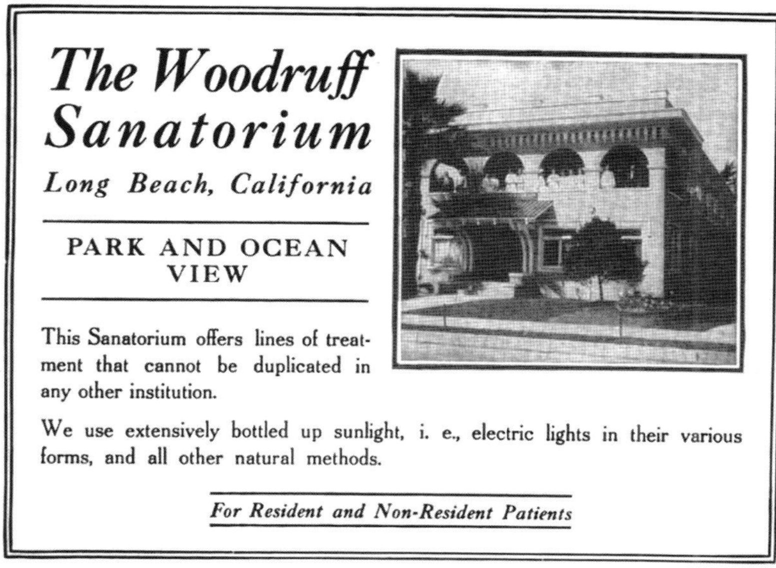

Above: Dr. W. L. Woodruff opened the Woodruff Sanatorium in 1905 at 137 Pacific Avenue. Woodruff specialized in "leucodescent light therapy" and "vibration" techniques. He vigorously opposed the vaccination of school children and led the fight against the city and state public health officers' orders. (*LBPL*)

Below: More than 60,000 people came to Long Beach for the 4th of July opening of the Pacific Electric trolley in 1902. The Los Angeles to Long Beach route ended at the corner of Ocean Park and Pacific avenues. The trolleys brought thousands to this seaside resort. Visitors came to see the newly built pier and auditorium as well as the "Walk of a Thousand Lights," a bowling alley, a bathhouse and the Majestic Skating rink.

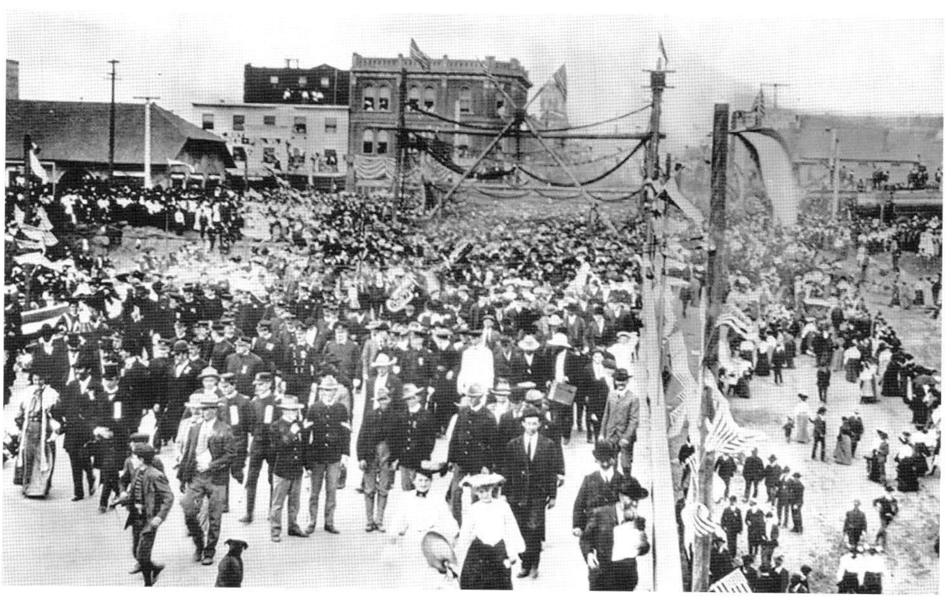

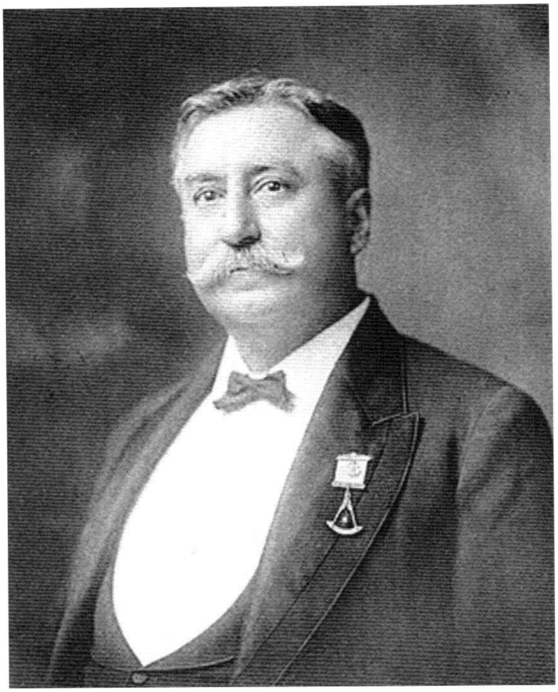

Long Beach physicians complained when their patients needed to be hospitalized, the trip to Los Angeles was "sometimes fraught with danger where the case is critical." A 1904 newspaper article announced that the city was planning a "large, modern, up-to-date hospital." The Long Beach Hospital Association was formed and hired local architect Harry F. Starbuck to design the facility which would be located at 10th Street and Linden Avenue. Starbuck designed many Long Beach buildings including the Masonic Temple and the United Presbyterian Church. (*HF*)

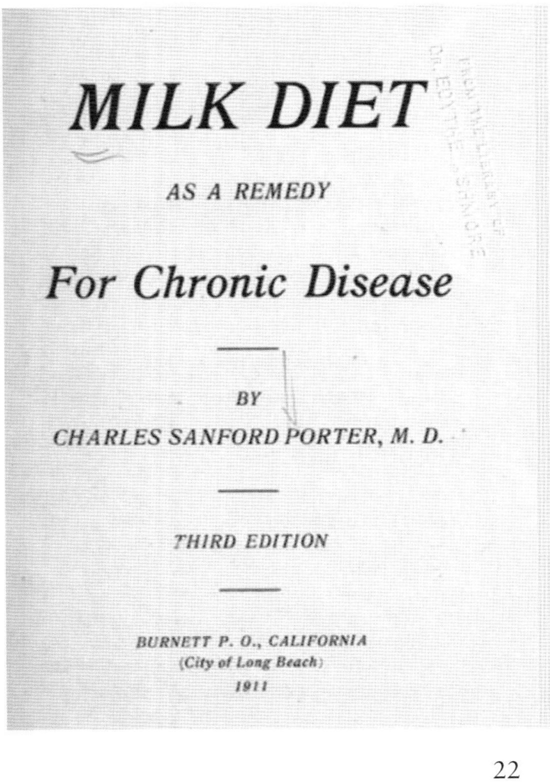

MILK DIET

AS A REMEDY

For Chronic Disease

BY

CHARLES SANFORD PORTER, M. D.

THIRD EDITION

BURNETT P. O., CALIFORNIA
(City of Long Beach)
1911

In 1905, Dr. Charles Porter authored the book, *Milk Diet as a Remedy for Chronic Disease*. He offered that a treatment of three weeks of raw milk, while sleeping on hair mattresses could cure most known diseases. In 1907, Porter opened the "Porter Milk Diet Sanitarium" at 737 Sunrise Boulevard, a location he advertised as "Burnett, California—two miles from Long Beach on the Salt Lake Railway and electric lines." Porter offered the "natural milk and rest cure" in "a quiet, homelike resting place." He opened another facility in Pasadena.

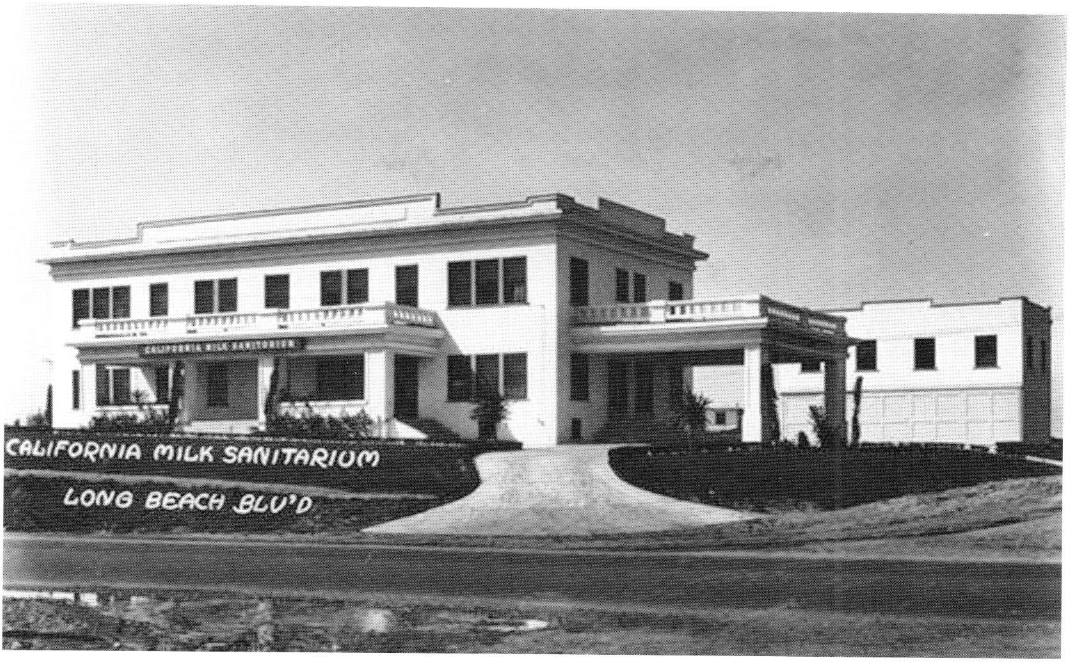

Milk diet and rest treatment facilities were popular for a time. The California Milk Sanitorium was operated by Aubrey Parks. It was located at 4010 American Avenue (now Long Beach Boulevard). Charles Porter closed his facility in 1924. (*LBPL*)

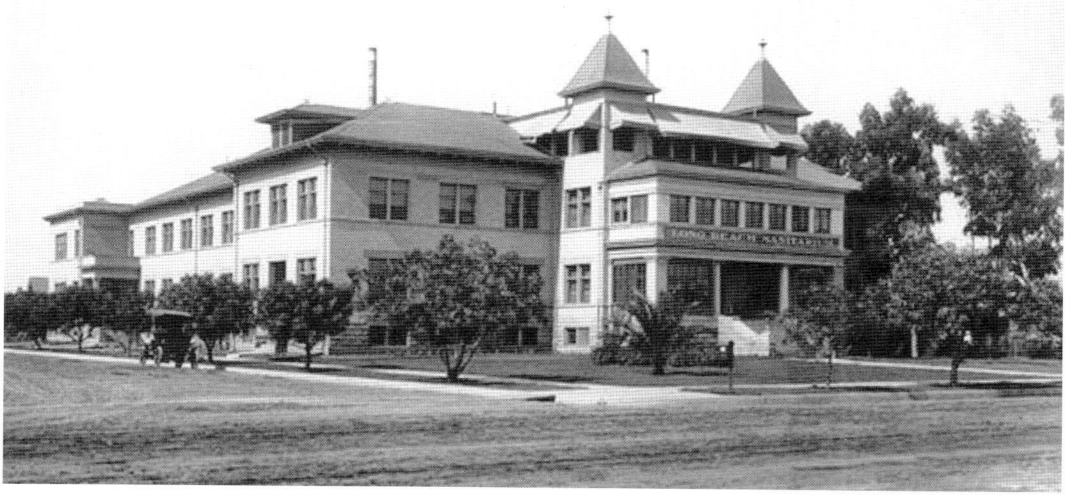

The Long Beach Hospital was staffed with local physicians and nurses. Miss Alice Hopkins was appointed the Nurse Matron for the hospital. Hopkins had served as a Nurse Matron in the county hospital. At the Long Beach Hospital, she quickly met with a staff rebellion when she discharged a nurse. The nurses told the Board of Directors they would all resign if Miss Hopkins was not fired for her "indiscretion." Hopkins left and took other nurses with her.

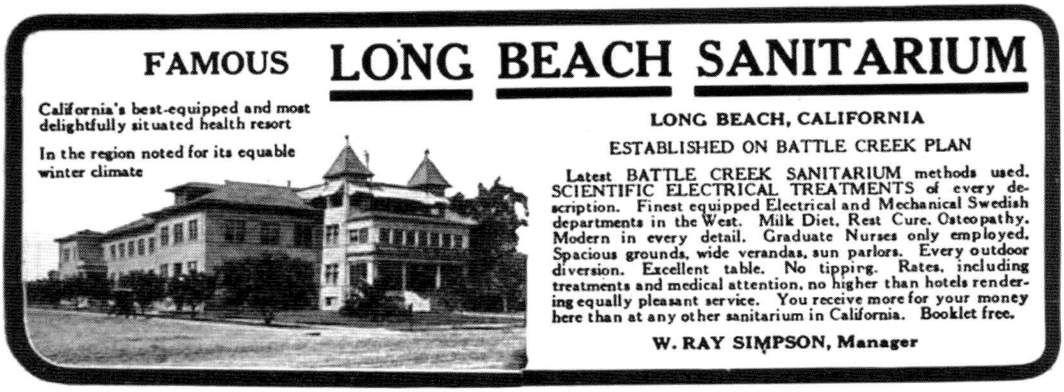
FAMOUS LONG BEACH SANITARIUM
California's best-equipped and most delightfully situated health resort
In the region noted for its equable winter climate
LONG BEACH, CALIFORNIA
ESTABLISHED ON BATTLE CREEK PLAN
Latest BATTLE CREEK SANITARIUM methods used. SCIENTIFIC ELECTRICAL TREATMENTS of every description. Finest equipped Electrical and Mechanical Swedish departments in the West. Milk Diet, Rest Cure, Osteopathy. Modern in every detail. Graduate Nurses only employed. Spacious grounds, wide verandas, sun parlors. Every outdoor diversion. Excellent table. No tipping. Rates, including treatments and medical attention, no higher than hotels rendering equally pleasant service. You receive more for your money here than at any other sanitarium in California. Booklet free.
W. RAY SIMPSON, Manager

In 1910, the building was purchased by W. Ray Simpson, who operated the facility with his physician wife, Abbie. Dr. Simpson had studied at the Battle Creek Sanitarium. Her husband advertised in numerous publications implying that the sanitarium was related to Battle Creek, even though it was not.

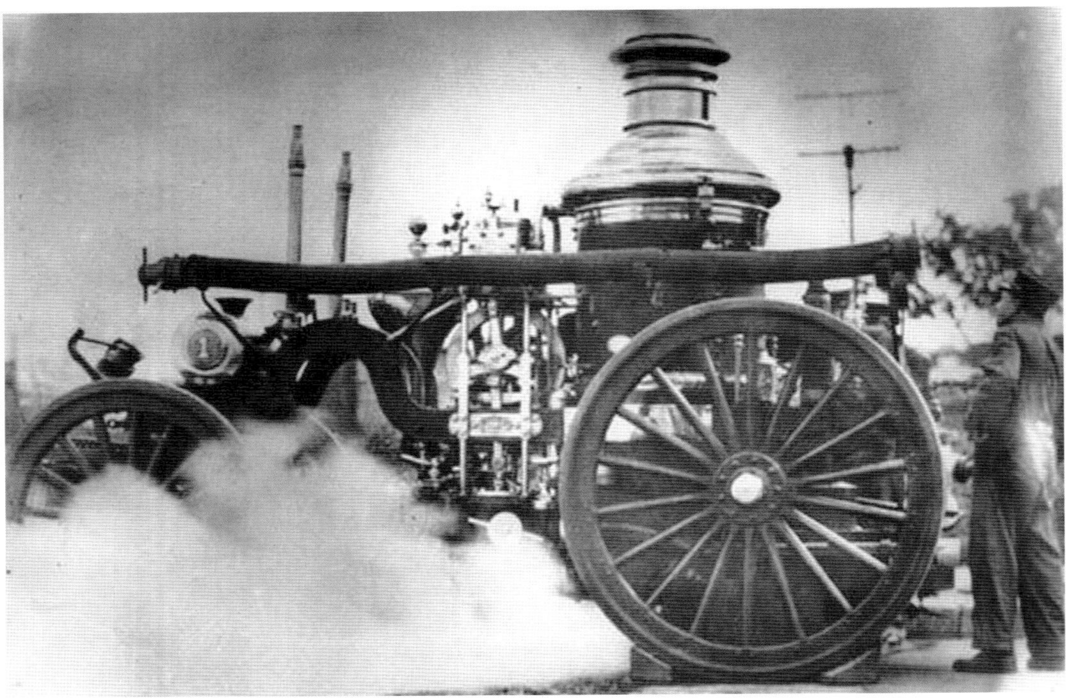

In 1913, the sanitarium caught fire due to oil drippings from the furnace. Twenty-three patients had to be removed through the "thick volumes of smoke." Because the sanitarium also served as a hospital, five surgical patients had to be transported on stretchers out of the building. Staff used an "emergency hose" to contain the fire until the Long Beach Fire Department responded. The fire was extinguished with reportedly little damage to the building. The Long Beach Public Library photo shows the fire department and apparatus in the early 1900s.

3

Seaside Memorial Hospital (1907-1960)

... the hospital is becoming more and more recognized as the place to go when one is ill.
Modern Hospital Vol 14, 1910

In 1907, a group of physicians met in the office of Dr. F. D. Bishop to discuss the incorporation of the Seaside Hospital Association of Long Beach. The following seventeen physicians and laymen were selected as its first board of directors: President, Dr. L. A. Perce; vice president, R. S. Oakford; secretary and treasurer, J. A. Miller; attorney, George A. Skinner. The other members of the board of directors are Drs. A. C. Sellery, H. O. Bates (first president of the Long Beach Medical Society), A. F. Hamman, F. L. Woodruff. E. R. Harvey, F. D. Bishop, E. M. Freeman, T. C. Donnell, J. H. Wood, J. M. Holden, W. Harriman Jones, W. F. Pascoe and E. H. Jackson.

The founders told local press, "the institution will be managed by physicians, among whom will be representative doctors of this city. Fine surgical work and expert nursing will be the specialties." The press noted, "the project is one of certain physicians who claim they have ignored in the present hospital and that conditions there are 'not satisfactory.'"

Drs. Harvey, Sellery and Bates were tasked with finding a suitable building. The committee had a difficult time getting city approval for a site on which to operate a hospital. When the committee selected a home at 519 Cedar Avenue, residents protested, and the council cancelled the permit. The Cedar location was to be leased from the owner, Mrs. I. B. Lambert, and would accommodate ten patients.

A site at Bishop Street and Independencia Avenue near Bixby and Carroll parks was also protested and the City Council rescinded that permit. The hospital was to be three stories and completed at a cost of $12,000. Local press accounts note that Seaside Hospital Association's projects were "nipped in the bud" eight times by the city council responding to resident protests.

A suitable location was found at the northwest corner of Broadway Street (then Railway) and Junipero Avenue. It was the former home of real estate magnate and Board of Education president, H. L. Enloe. New furnishings were added, and the hospital opened with twelve rooms.

In 1910, the Seaside Hospital Association proposed erecting "a larger modern hospital building of twenty-two rooms" at the corner of St. James Avenue and Loma Vista Drive, which was located on the "lowlands between Long Beach and San Pedro." The council failed to give a permit.

Two lots of farmland were finally purchased in 1913 from Steven Townsend, a local realtor. Coincidently, Townsend lived at 504 Cedar Avenue, just steps away from 519 Cedar where Seaside was first planned to be located.

Later, Townsend joined the Seaside Hospital Association Board of Directors. Physicians raised $30,000 for construction of a thirty-one-room hospital. Jess Jones, an architect with offices at 501 Termino Avenue, designed the hospital, located at 14th Street and Magnolia Avenue. The hospital expanded several times and in 1937, the Board of Directors reincorporated as "Seaside Memorial Hospital." Seaside's bed capacity went from twelve to 427 by the 1940s.

In 1918, Mary K. West was appointed superintendent of the new nurses' training school at Seaside. Because of the influenza epidemic, the school was turned into patient wards. It was officially opened in 1919 with twenty-one students. The school was a three-year, residential program. Graduate nurses could either remain at Seaside or seek employment as private duty nurses. Nursing developed as a profession when more than 10,000 nurses served during World War I (1914-1918).

Long Beach was quickly becoming an industrial town as well as seaside resort because of its port and the presence of the U.S. Navy. Seaside Hospital took care of patients who were victims of accidents caused by horses, trolleys, automobiles, oil explosions, electricity, poison, shotguns and knives, and botched abortions.

In 1931, bones of several mastodons were uncovered while making brick in the old brickyard north of Seaside Hospital. Bones of the "imperial elephant" were also found at Spring Street and Orange Avenue, Spring Street and Cherry Avenue, 36th and Walnut Avenue, and 37th and Atlantic Avenue.

The 1933 earthquake severely damaged Seaside Hospital (and St. Mary's Hospital). Several areas flooded, and walls crumbled. Dr. Sterling Pillsbury was in the process of delivering a baby when the tremblor struck. He pushed the delivery table to a safe corner and saved both baby and mother.

During WWII, Seaside became the largest military hospital in the area until it was replaced by the U.S. Naval Hospital on 7th Street. In 1942, Seaside was awarded $71,000 for construction by the Federal Works Agency for needed expansion. By 1947, the hospital had 427 beds and operated five community clinics.

In 1949, the Carnation Milk Company and the Long Beach Hospitals United group ran full-page newspaper ads asking residents to pray that city councilmen would vote to fund 14 million dollars in city bonds to repair local hospitals and to increase the number of hospital beds. The City Council did approve the bonds on the condition the hospitals turned over their deeds to the city. Only St. Mary's Hospital did not participate.

The City of Long Beach is the site of one of the largest oil and gas fields in the U.S. When oil was extracted from the "tidelands area," the state fought for ownership rights and the revenues from the oil and gas. In 1955, the State Supreme Court ruled that Long Beach could only use tidelands oil revenues in tidelands areas and not for general fund projects. The ruling killed the city's promise to use this oil and gas revenue to fund: $16 million for hospitals, $3.7 million for parks and $400,000 for four branch libraries. Voters approved a 10.6-million-dollar bond issue which was distributed to several hospitals.

As the military expanded in Long Beach, so did the number of babies. Seaside boasted that between 1945 and 1953, more than 14,500 babies were born without a single maternal death.

On June 12, 1960, Richard Leland Feld was the last baby born at Seaside Memorial Hospital. His cry was sent over the telephone and triggered motors that opened the doors of the new Memorial Hospital located at 2180 E. Atlantic Avenue. The city provided an initial 6.5 million dollars in bonds. The land was owned by the City and located in a blighted area. The site was selected because it was "the geographic center of the city" and allowed additional buildings and easy access to the freeways. Most importantly, it provided "a good view of the city and the winds keep the area free from smog."

The 11-million-dollar, 400-bed hospital officially opened on June 25, 1960, and was touted as the "first space-age hospital." It was built of reinforced concrete in the shape of a cross and named Memorial Hospital of Long Beach. Today, it is known as Memorial Medical Center and part of the Memorial Health Care system based in Fountain Valley, California.

The old Seaside Hospital was sold to Los Angeles County for 1.6 million dollars and renamed "El Cerrito Hospital." It was utilized as a facility for "oldsters with chronic illnesses." Eventually, it became El Cerrito Health Out-Patient Center and then finally the Long Beach Comprehensive Care Center, which today provides outpatient health care services to low-income residents.

In 1907, Seaside Hospital was opened in a private home located at the northwest corner of Railway (Broadway) and Junipero. It offered sixteen beds and was staffed by many of the physicians and nurses who had worked at the Long Beach Hospital. Miss Ida Stafford was named as the nurse superintendent of the hospital in 1908. Nurse superintendents were the first hospital administrators. (*LBPL*)

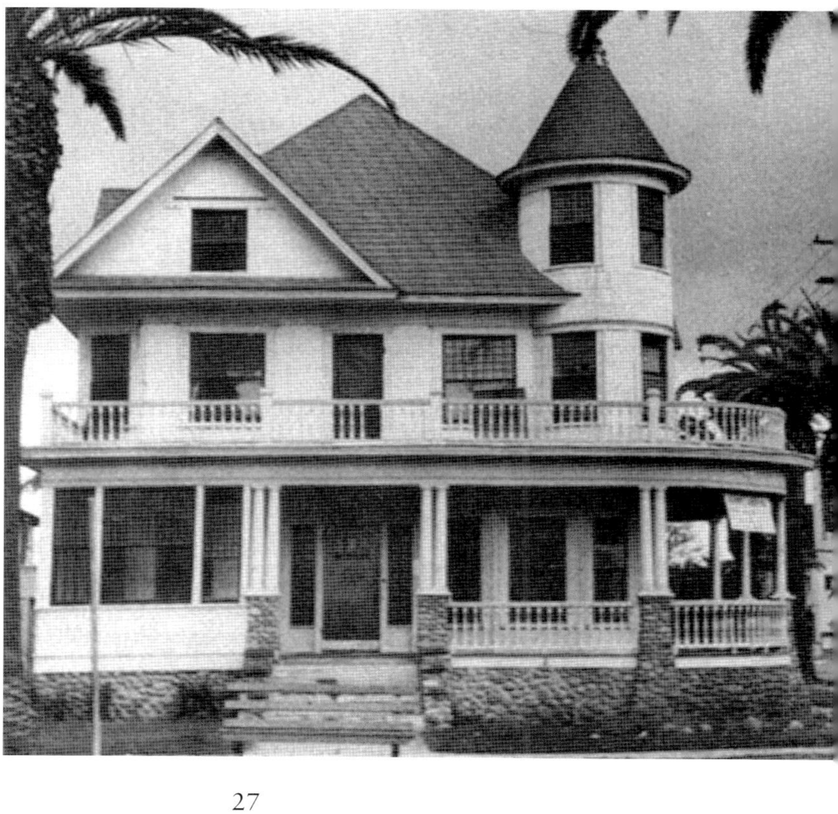

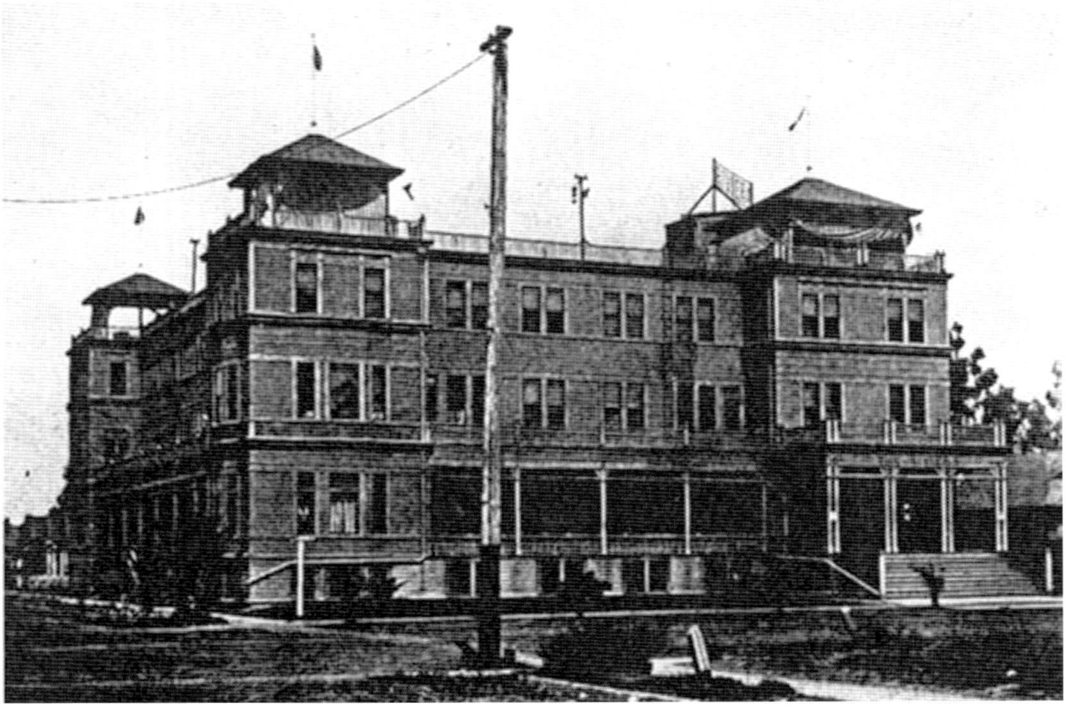

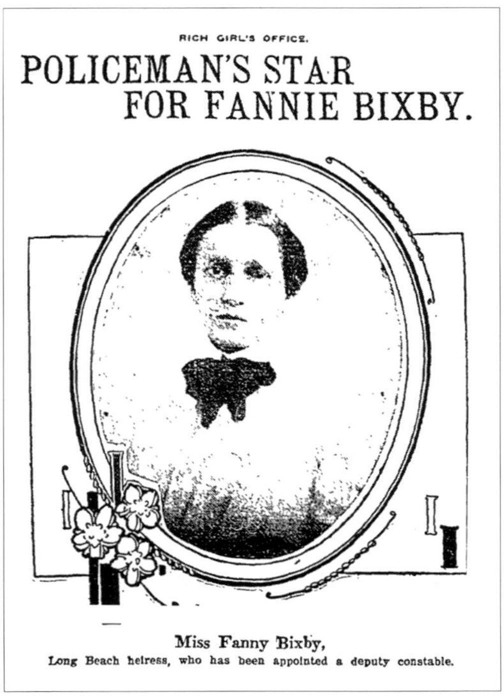

RICH GIRL'S OFFICE.

POLICEMAN'S STAR FOR FANNIE BIXBY.

Miss Fanny Bixby,

Long Beach heiress, who has been appointed a deputy constable.

Above: Although the population of Long Beach was only 16,000 in 1910, six facilities were listed in the city directory as "hospital" or "sanitarium": The Bishop Hospital, Long Beach Sanitarium, Pacific Avenue Sanitarium, Porter Sanitarium, Schutz Sanitarium (pictured) and Seaside Hospital.

Left: A school of nursing was opened at Seaside in 1918 and headed by Ida Stafford. Stafford was a close friend of Fannie Bixby, the last daughter of Jotham and Margaret Bixby. Fannie was a suffragist and social activist. She served as the city's first female police constable.

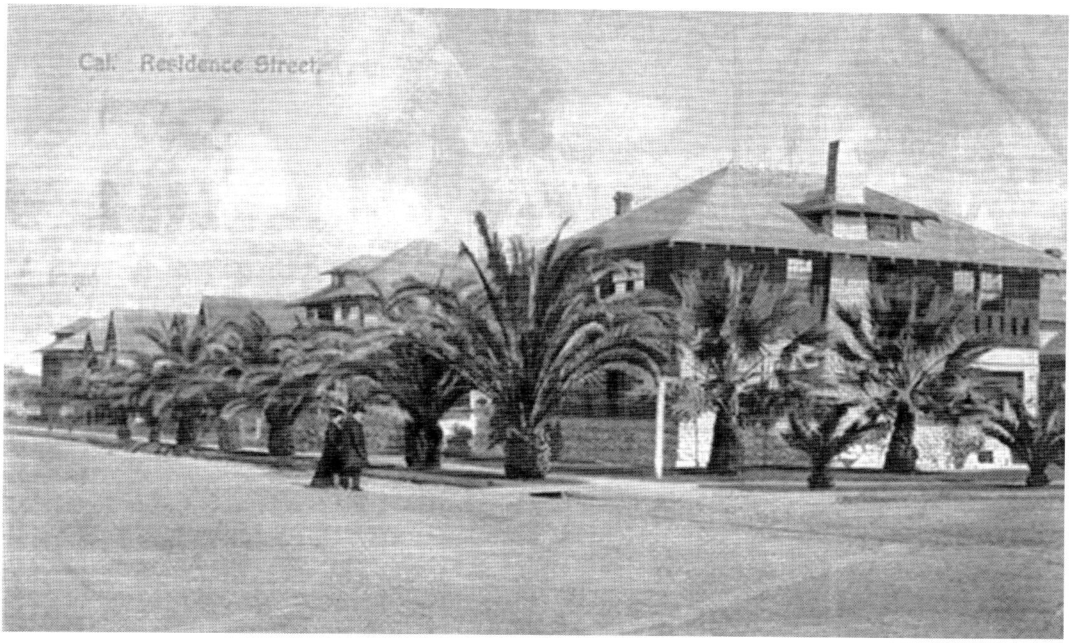

In 1913, two farm lots were purchased from Stephen Townsend (pictured) near Magnolia Avenue and 14th Street for the new Seaside Hospital. Townsend, who came to Long Beach in 1895, was a prominent real estate developer and instrumental in the establishment of a port of Long Beach. His home at 504 Cedar Avenue (pictured) was just steps away from 519 Cedar which had been considered for the first site of Seaside. When residents objected to a hospital in their neighborhood, the City Council rejected the permit.

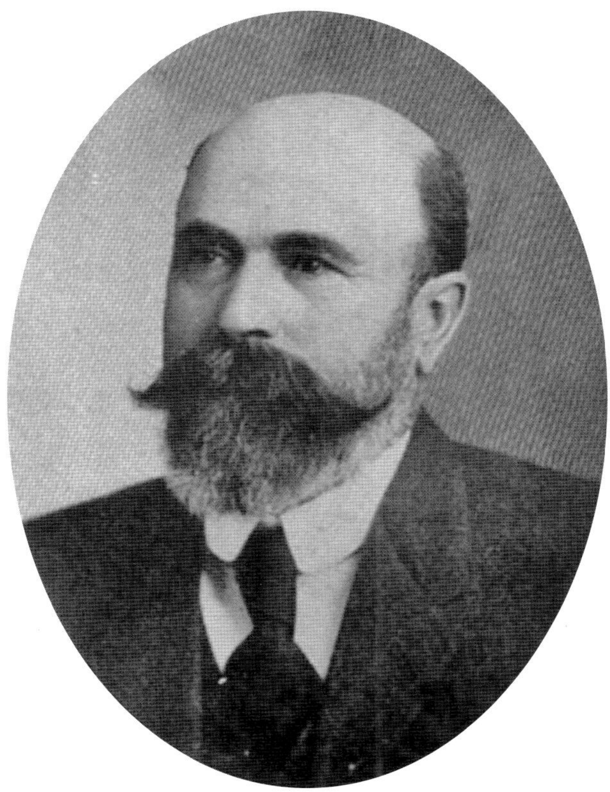

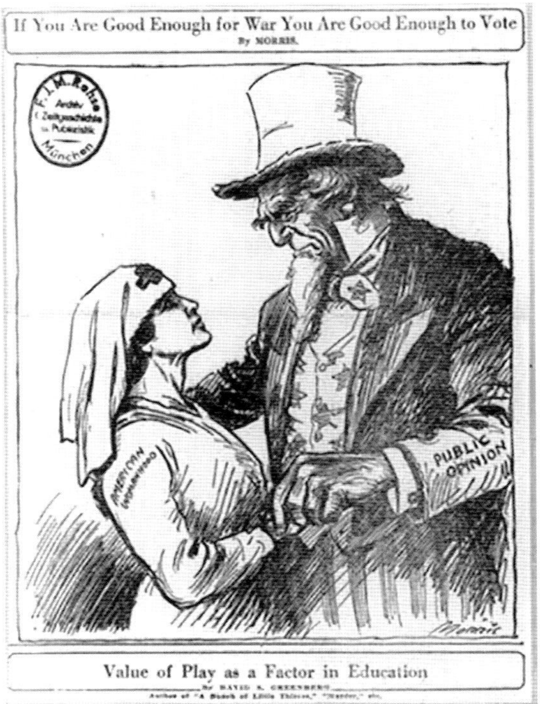
If You Are Good Enough for War You Are Good Enough to Vote
By MORRIS.
PUBLIC OPINION
Value of Play as a Factor in Education

Left: Nursing programs were of three years in length and provided hospitals and sanitariums with a live-in workforce. WWI utilized thousands of nurses which aided in the call for suffrage for women. Posters showing nurses tending wounded soldiers posed the question of "why can't she have the ballot?" Women won the right to vote in 1920. (*LOC*)

Below: As the city grew, so did the need for hospitalization. A larger two-story annex was added to Seaside in 1921 at the cost of $165,000.

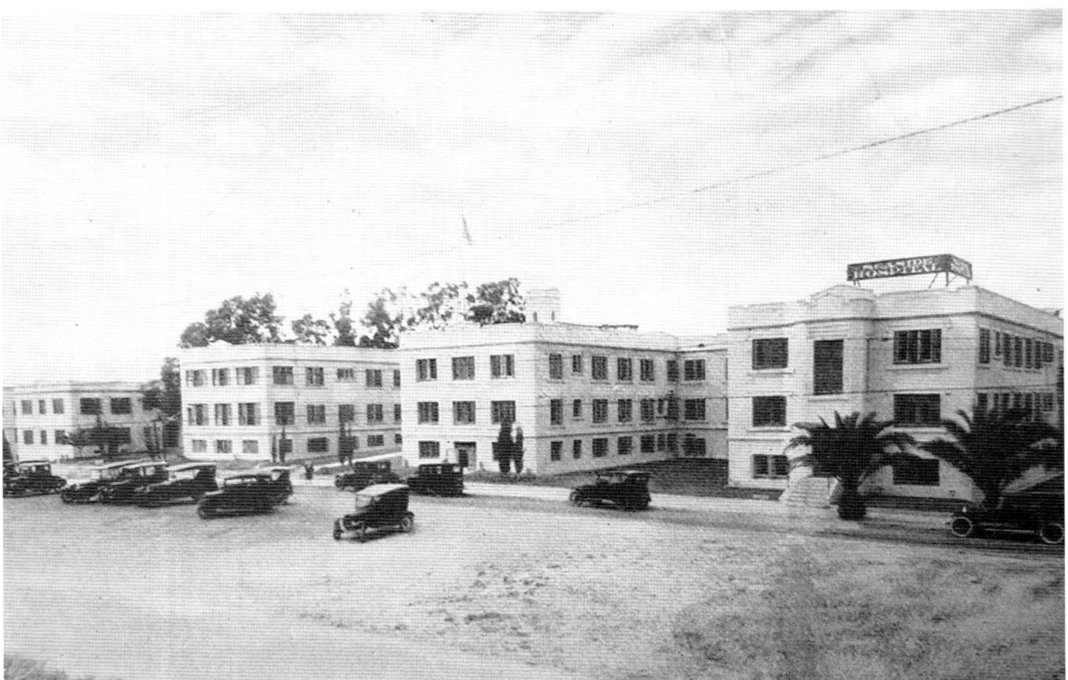

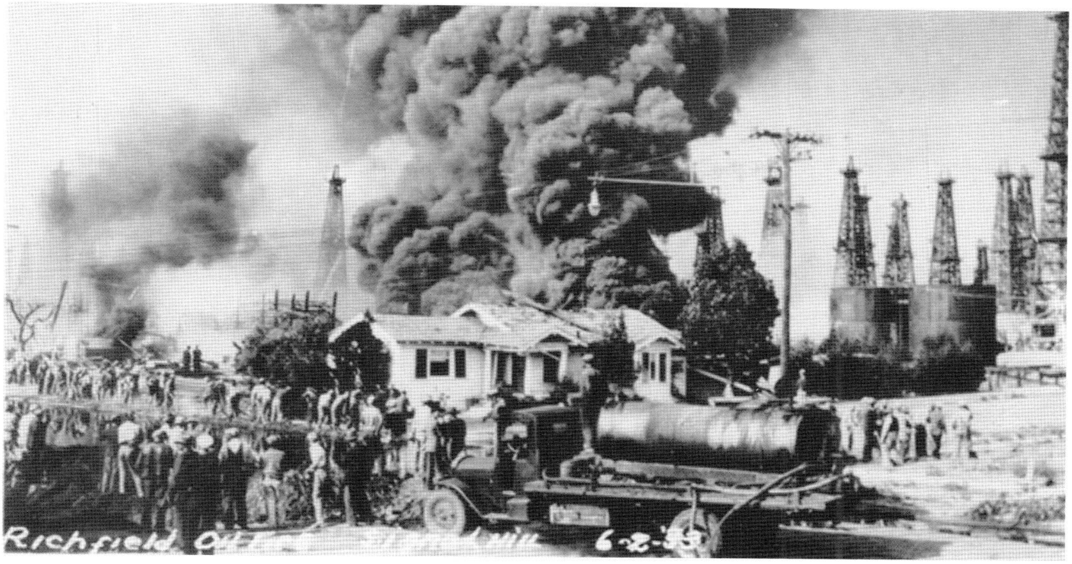

Automobiles, trolleys, oil refineries and other industrial areas were the cause of many horrible accidents that provided patients for Seaside. The Richfield Oil Company refinery explosion in June 1933 killed seventeen and brought dozens to the hospital for treatment. The blast from the oil refinery could be felt thirty miles away. (*CL*)

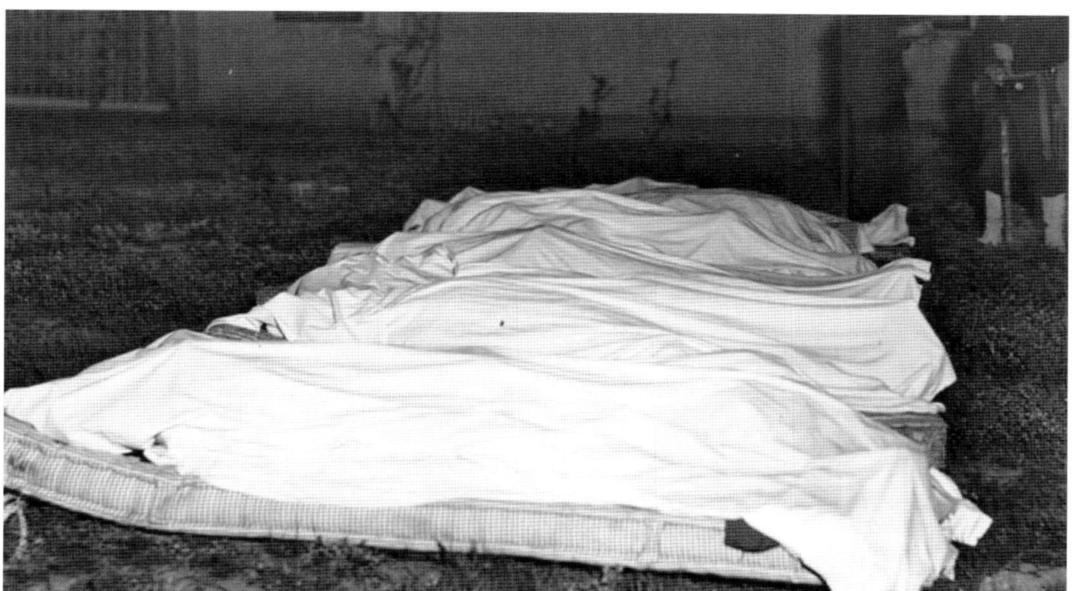

Earlier in 1933, Long Beach was hit by a major earthquake. Seaside, like many buildings and schools in the city, sustained considerable damage. Bodies were placed behind the hospital out of public view. It would take several years before the hospital was fully repaired. (*USGS*)

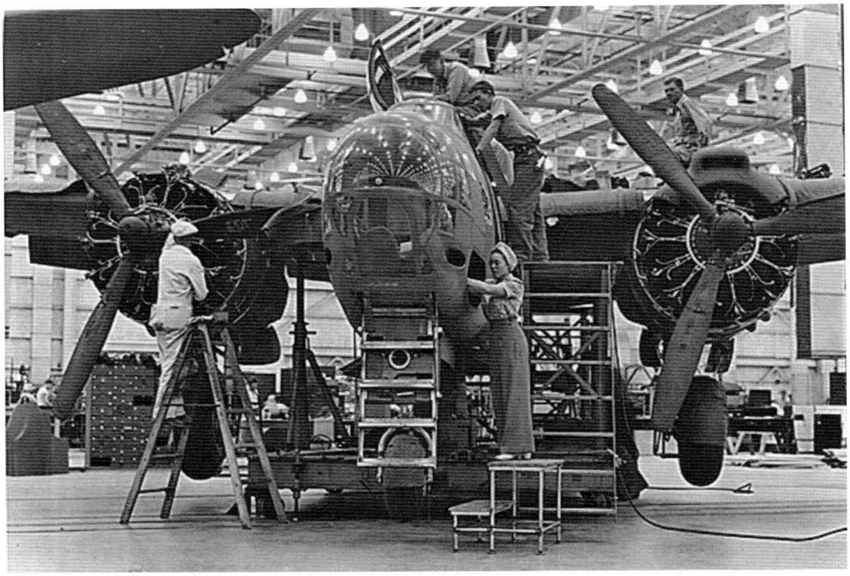

Above: For many years, Long Beach was a home port to the U.S. Navy. Its airport was utilized as an Army airfield. Douglas Aircraft (and the women who worked there) produced the planes that helped win World War II. (*LOC*)

Below: From the 1940s, physicians and others called for a new hospital. In 1949, the Carnation Company and Emergency Citizens Committee of the Long Beach Hospitals United funded full-page ads calling on residents to "pray" that the city council would approve $14 million dollars in bonds to repair and expand local hospitals. A survey had been commissioned that resulted in a finding that the area needed 929 more hospital beds. Under the bond scenario, the city would hold title to the hospitals and lease them back for one dollar a year.

THIS VOICE CAN NOT BE STILLED! HOPE CAN NOT BE SMOTHERED!

The danger point in any movement for civic betterment comes when the proponents of worthy causes falter under the fire of opposition. Angry words, blind antagonism and closed minds have caused many noble plans for the good of the people to perish.

In answer to the countless telephone inquiries and letters from the people of Long Beach, it can be stated that the Emergency Citizens Committee for Long Beach Hospitals United will not be diverted from its duty to the community.

The urgency of the hospital situation here does not permit a single person in the community to shrink back a single inch in the face of the feeble criticism which has arisen.

With renewed vigor, we will continue to tell the story of our city's critical hospital plight.

We will continue to tell it—honestly and fairly—in the future, as we have in the past.

We ask only that you keep an open mind.

Soon the entire story will be told.

And YOU will be the judge and jury!

Charges of "emotionalism!" have been hurled at the medical men and distinguished civic-leaders who have asked City Council to authorize a bond issue of $14,000,000 for additional hospital facilities for Seaside Memorial Hospital, Community Hospital and Long Beach Osteopathic Hospital.

Upland Oil Revenue, however, can no longer, by Charter Amendment of 1942, be used for any purpose other than general bonds and general purposes of the city.

All other bonds of the city—water, gas, harbor—are retired out of the funds of those three departments and no upland millions whatsoever can be used for the water, gas and harbor bond indebtedness.

Since the early part of May, 1949 — last month — upland oil revenue must be diverted to the general purpose fund of the city inasmuch as all general bond requirements have been met and the money set aside. This money must be used for general purposes of the city until such time as there may be other general city bonds outstanding at which time upland oil revenue again will be designated for the redemption of such bonds.

It was in the early part of May, 1949—last month—that the upland fund had accumulated $13,232,230.00, providing for the ultimate retirement of the last of all general bonds.

Thus it was in May—last month—that the upland money became available for the first time for the general purposes and the welfare of the city and its people.

From July 1, 1949 to June 30, 1950 upland oil will produce $2,030,310 for the city treasury, according to the official estimate of the petroleum engineers of the Long Beach Harbor Department.

Throughout all the years to come the upland oil millions belong to You, The People of Long Beach.

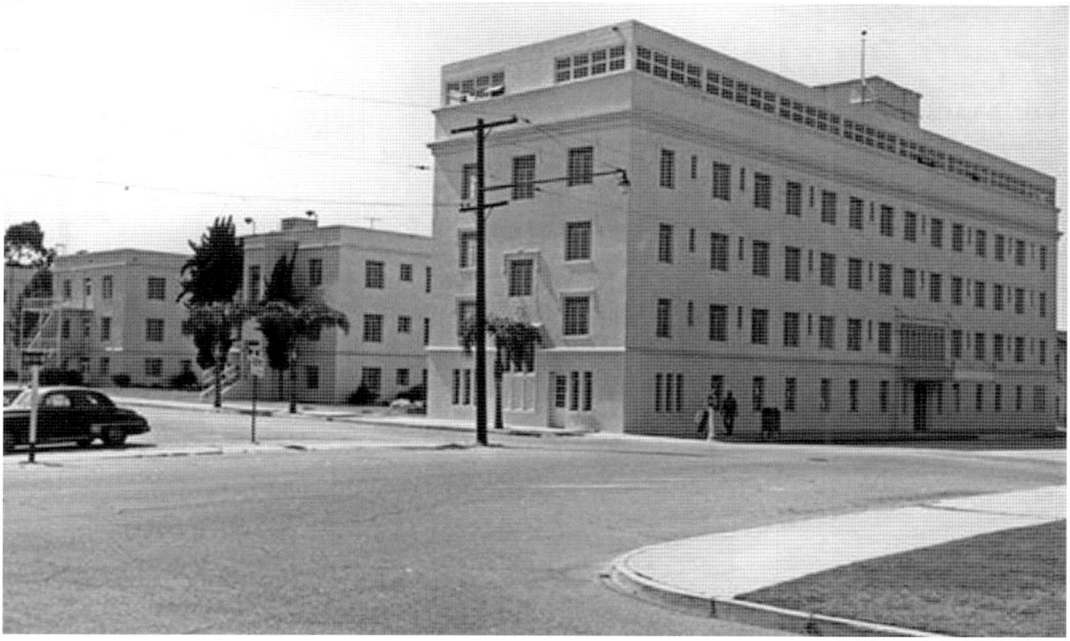

By the late 1950s, Seaside Hospital included several buildings and was known as Seaside Memorial Hospital. More than 14,500 babies were born at Seaside between 1945-1953 without a single maternal death. Additional newspaper advertisements were taken out by the "Auxiliary to the Children's Memorial Hospital," a group formed to promote a children's hospital at the new Seaside Memorial Hospital. The group advocated for a specialty hospital because of the polio scare.

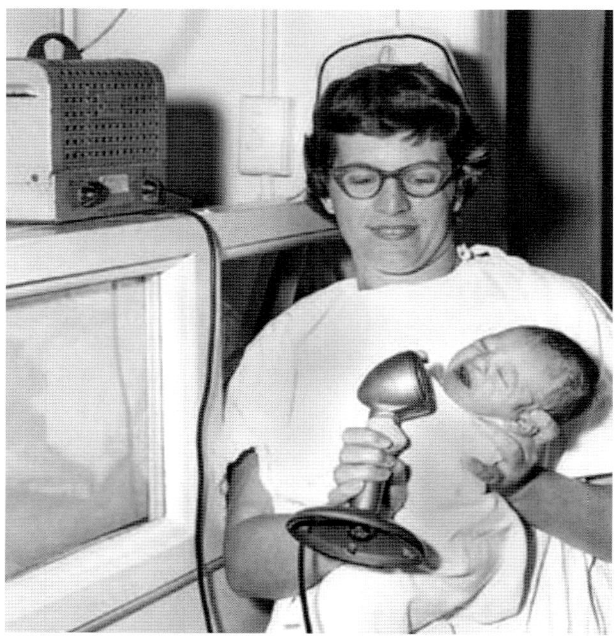

On June 12, 1960, the cry of a newborn baby boy, Richard Leland Feld, was sent over telephone lines to trigger motors which opened the doors to the newly constructed Memorial Hospital of Long Beach. (*MC*)

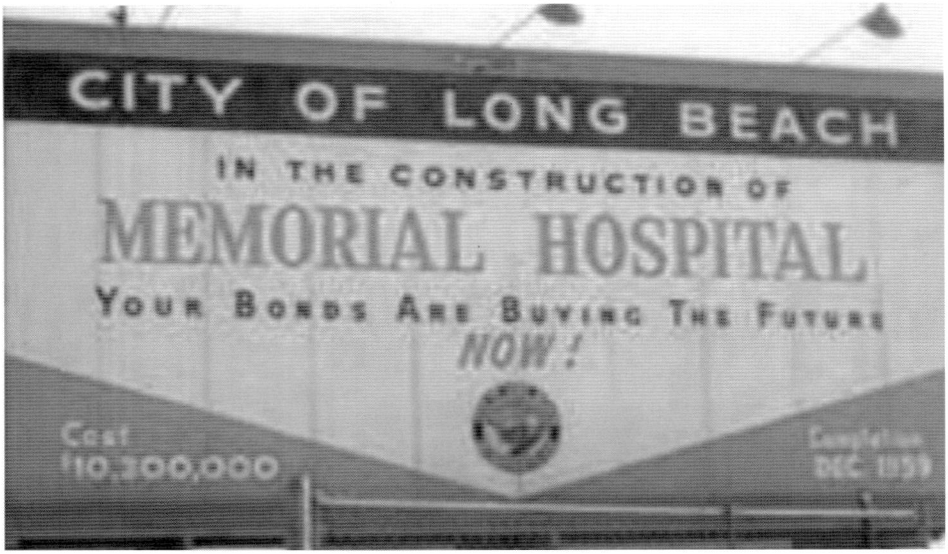
CITY OF LONG BEACH
IN THE CONSTRUCTION OF
MEMORIAL HOSPITAL
YOUR BONDS ARE BUYING THE FUTURE
NOW!

The hospital was constructed for 11 million dollars, including 6.5 million dollars in city bonds. The 400-bed facility featured twelve operating rooms, 802 employees and 448 physicians on staff. (*MC*)

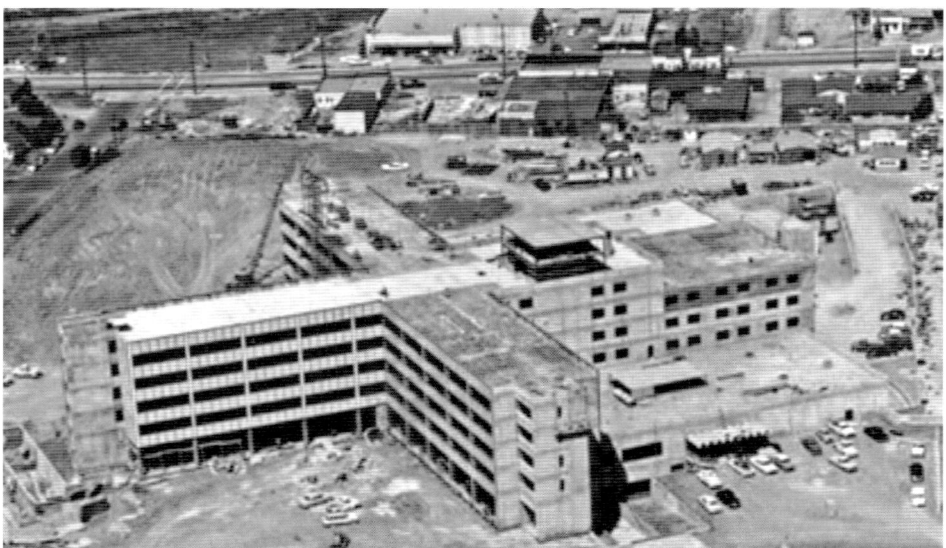

The hospital was called "the first space-age hospital" because of its design and use of reinforced concrete. It was designed in the shape of a cross by architects: Jess Jones, William Lockett, R. L., Poper, Hugh Gibbs and Kenneth Wing. J. C. Boespflug was the contractor and Maris Bergson designed the interior. The city financed the hospital on land that was in the most blighted area of Long Beach. When completed, the city touted that the location was perfect because it had "easy access to freeways and a good view of the city." (*MC*)

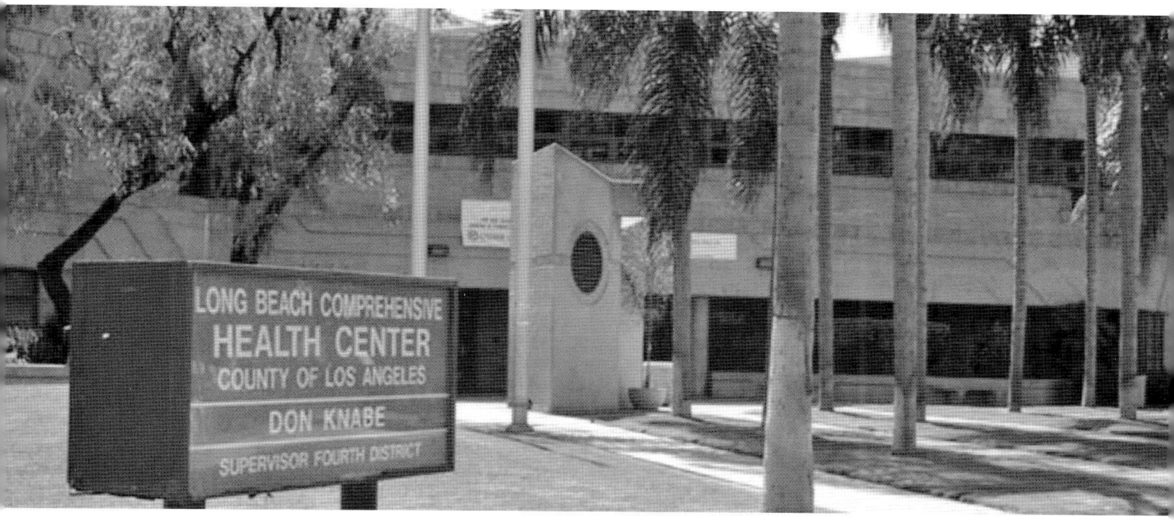

Above: Two hundred and nine patients, including six premature born babies, were transferred from the old Seaside site to the new Memorial Hospital at 2801 Atlantic Avenue. Members of fourteen local labor unions assisted in the move for free. The old Seaside Hospital became a LA County facility and was renamed El Cerrito Hospital. It later was renamed Los Angeles Comprehensive Health Center and continues to provide healthcare to low-income patients. (*LAC*)

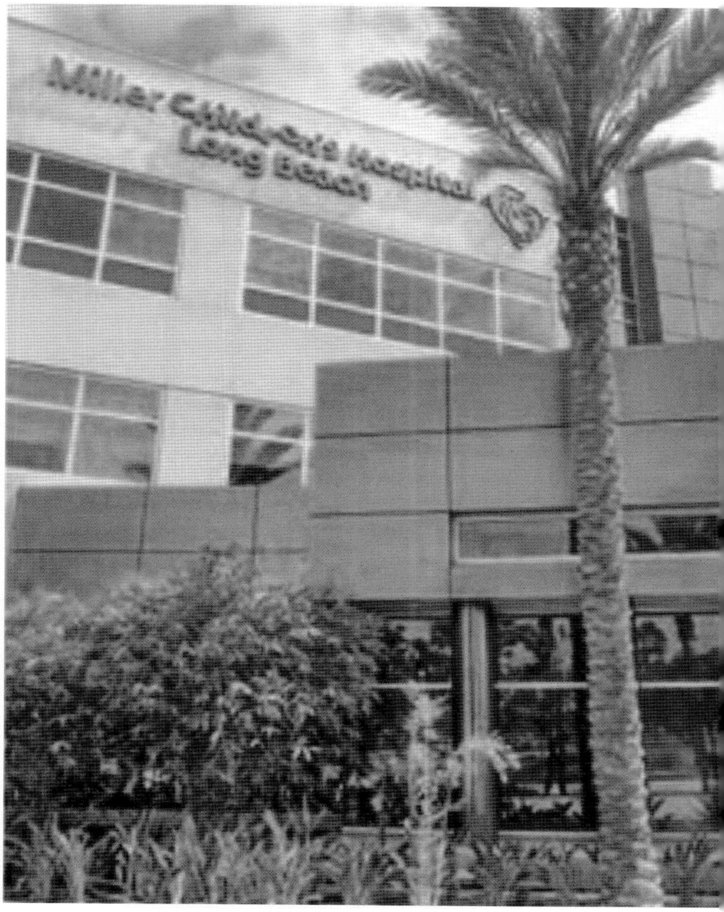

Right: Today, Memorial Medical Center includes Miller Children's Hospital and the Children's Clinic. Memorial Medical Center in Long Beach is part of the Memorial Healthcare system based in Fountain Valley, California. (*MC*)

4

St. Mary's Hospital of Long Beach (1923-1975)

A life for God; a heart for others

From Sisters of Charity of the Incarnate Word

It took time for the Catholic church to gain a foothold in Long Beach. By the early 1900s, most Christian denominations had established churches in the city. However, there were accounts some residents publicly opposed the building of a Catholic church.

Land was purchased at the corner of Sixth Street and Olive Avenue and on September 16, 1902, ground was broken for St Anthony's Catholic Church. The first Catholic school opened in 1916. By 1922, there were over 2,000 members of the parish. A second Catholic Church—St. Matthew's—was built at Temple Avenue and 7th Street. In 1926, there were three other Catholic churches added to Long Beach.

When Dr. Truman Boyd announced he wanted to sell the sanitarium at 10th Street and Linden Avenue, St. Anthony's parish priest, Fr. John M. Hegarty, contacted the Sisters of Charity of the Incarnate Word in Houston, asking that they purchase the facility and start a Catholic hospital.

The Sisters of Charity of the Incarnate Word had been established in France and a small group came to Texas after the Civil War. The Sisters focused on providing healthcare and helping communities survive devastating hurricanes and a smallpox epidemic.

The Sisters were offered several alternatives for financing the building. They purchased the sanitarium and refurbished it into seventy-bed St. Mary's Hospital Long Beach. It opened in 1923 with Dr. Truman Boyd as its first "chief of staff" and Mother Elizabeth O'Neill as its first administrator.

The Catholic community raised funds for a larger hospital. When the depression hit, plans were put on hold. The 1933 earthquake destroyed the original hospital, convent and chapel. One of the remaining stucco buildings was converted into a temporary hospital in which earthquake victims were treated.

In 1937, a new fire- and earthquake-proof St. Mary's Hospital opened. The four-story structure was designed by I. E. Loveless. Throughout WWII, the hospital was full. Finally, in 1946, St. Mary's received a federal Hill-Burton grant for expansion. Unlike several of the local hospitals, St. Mary's refused to sign over its deed to get funds from the city and raised building funds on its own.

St. Mary's Hospital broke ground in 1947 for a six-story, 2-million-dollar addition. By 1949, the hospital featured 275 beds and seventy-five bassinets. Medical staff performed several medical "firsts" in Long Beach in the 1950s: first cardiac-catheterization (1955), first artificial kidney treatment (1959) and the first open-heart surgery using a heart pump (1959).

Once again, St. Mary Hospital expanded with a five story "east wing." In 1962, there were 349 beds and cardiac, emergency, respiratory and maternity units. The hospital reported 10,000 emergency room visits and 3,000 births. In 1965, Medicare and Medicaid became law and local hospitals needed additional beds and services for the elderly and poor.

St. Mary's continued to grow and in 1970 added the Bauer Hospital. This 10-million-dollar project grew to 15 million dollars and boosted the number of beds to 550. St. Mary's Hospital officially became St. Mary Medical Center on December 3, 1975. Today, it serves as one of two trauma centers in the City and provides numerous community health-care services in the central area of the City. St. Mary Medical Center was the first health-care organization in Long Beach to provide care and treatment to persons with AIDs.

Founders of Saint Anthony Parish

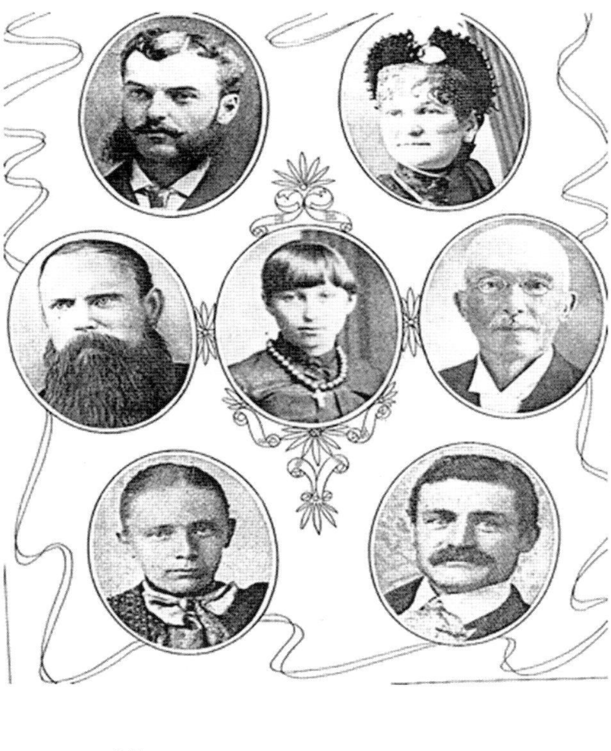

It would take a non-Catholic, Mrs. John Morris, to organize the first fundraising project that led to the construction of St. Anthony's Catholic Church on two acres of donated land at 6th Street and Olive Avenue. In 1902, ground was broken, and Father Ramon Ferrer was appointed as first pastor. *(SACH)*

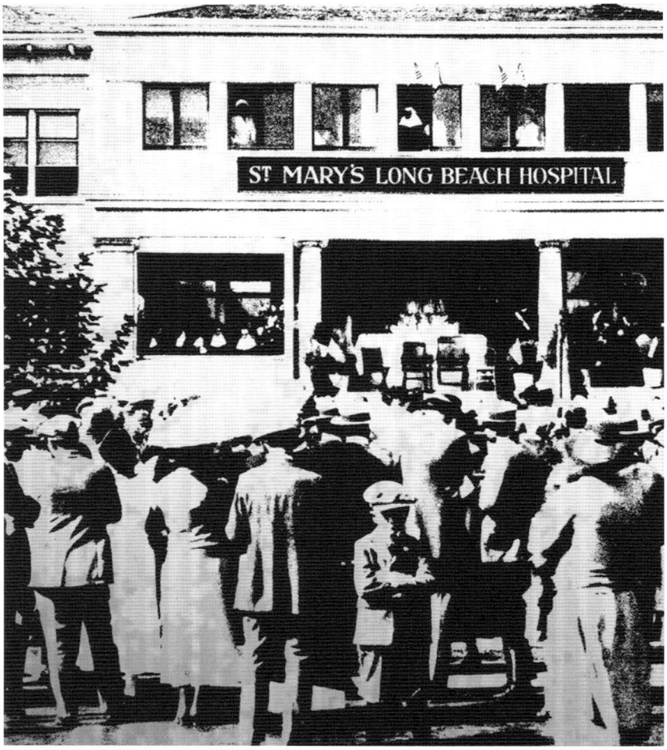

Left: The Sisters of Charity of the Incarnate Word agreed to purchase the sanitarium, and in the spring of 1923, they paid $160,000. They refurbished it and opened a seventy-bed hospital by August 1. Sister. M. Elizabeth O'Neill was named as the first administrator. At city Hall, residents and councilmembers continued advocating for a community hospital now that city had a private hospital (Seaside) and a Catholic hospital. (*SMMCH*)

Below: In 1914, a new St. Anthony's church was constructed. Like most buildings in Long Beach, it was constructed of brick. When the 1933 earthquake hit, the church was destroyed. (*SACH*)

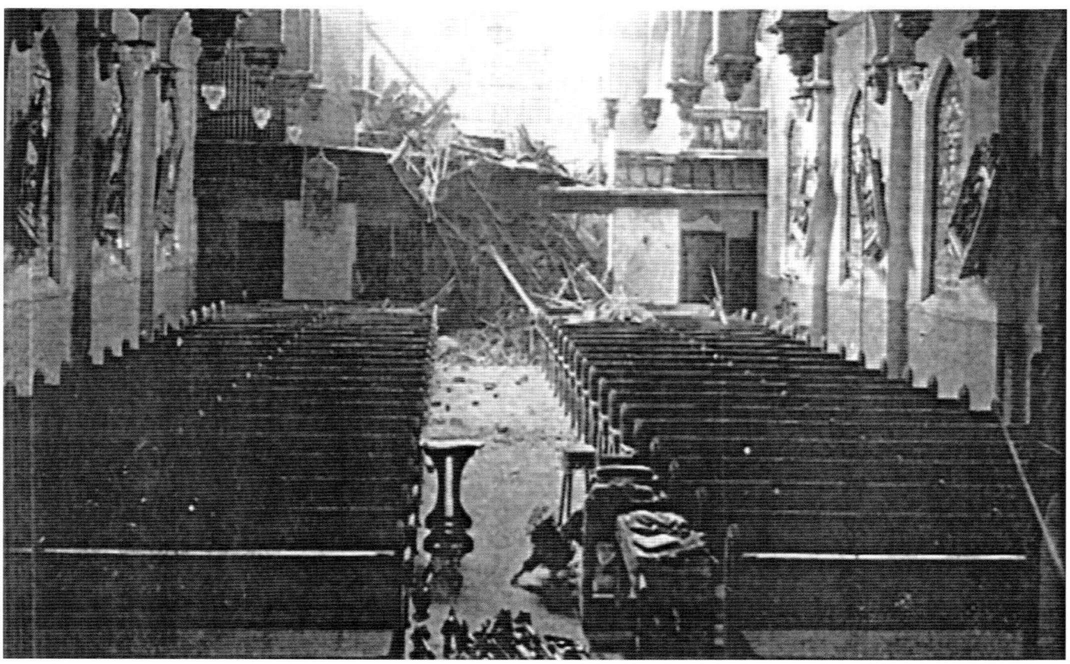

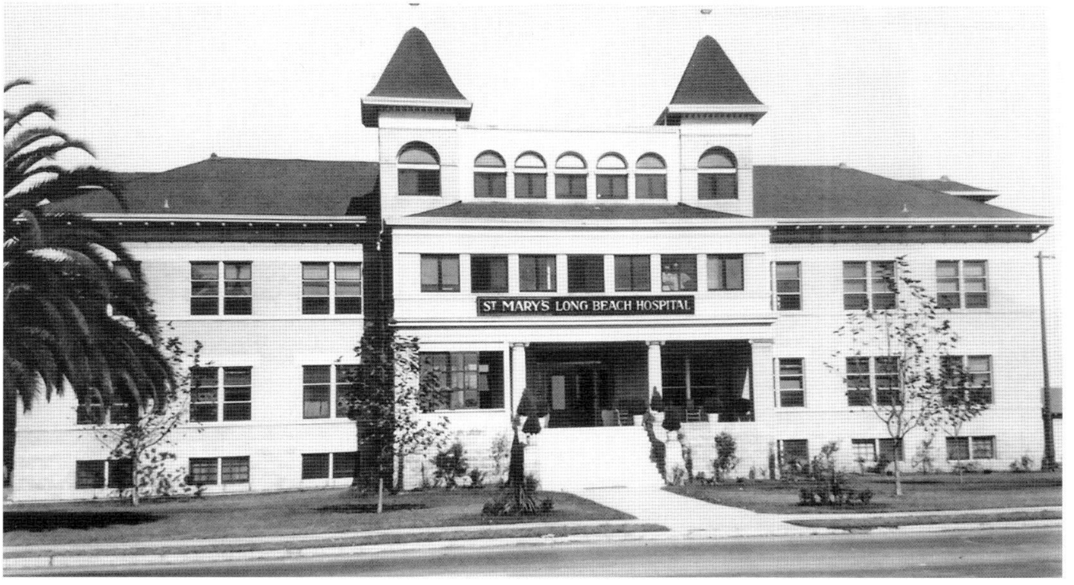

Above and below: The hospital, chapel and convent of St. Mary's Hospital of Long Beach were destroyed by the 1933 earthquake. The Sisters converted a remaining stucco building into a hospital with twenty-five beds. It took over four years to rebuild a new hospital. (*LBPL*)

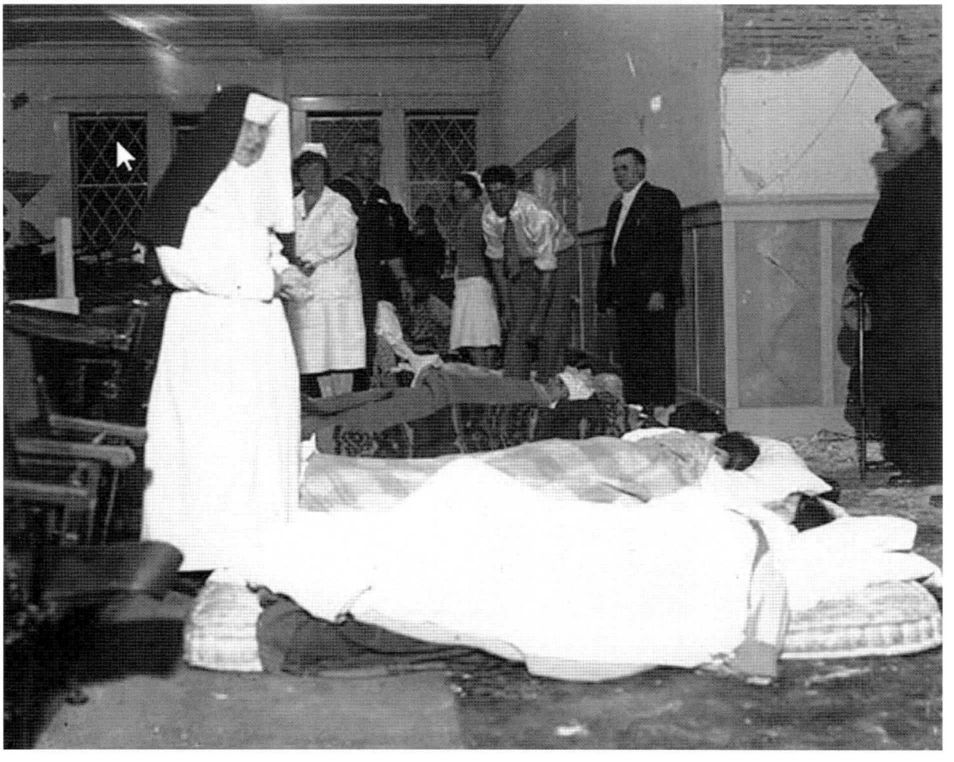

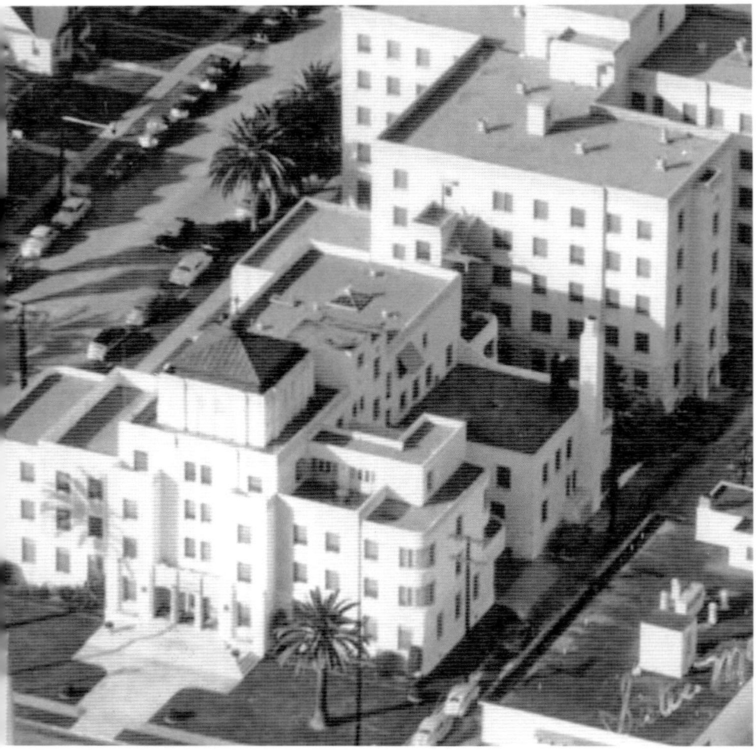

In 1937, St. Mary's Hospital constructed a new building to replace the one damaged by earthquake. The building was earthquake and fire proof. In 1949, a six-story, 2-million-dollar expansion north of the frontage was completed, bringing bed capacity to 253 beds. (*SMMCH*)

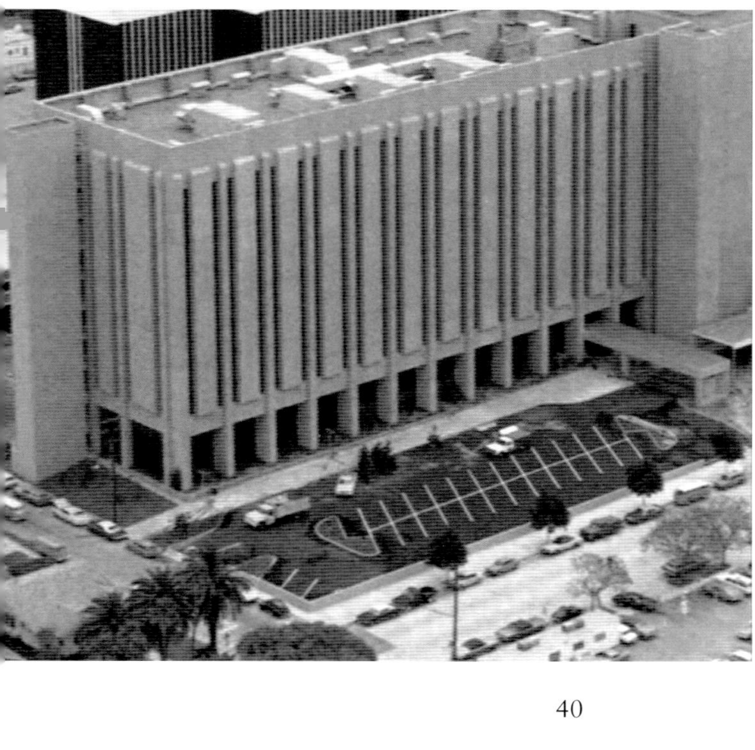

As the city expanded, so did St. Mary's Hospital. In May 1962, St. Mary Hospital raised 1.3 million dollars in donations and constructed a new five-story East Wing, bringing bed capacity to 349. On October 18, 1970, ground was broken for a 10-million-dollars project, funded in a great part (4 million dollars) by Modestus and Evalyn Bauer. It added 230 new beds, including sixty beds for intensive care. (*SMMCH*)

5

RESIDENTS WANT A "PEOPLE'S HOSPITAL"

> In my three years residence here, I have learned to love California and Californians, but existing selfishness and opposition in reference to hospitals would disgrace darkest Africa.
>
> Letter to editor by Fillmore Condit, 1920

In 1914, the Women's City Club declared a great need for a "maternity and detention hospital" and called upon the city to "secure $60,000 in bonds for its immediate establishment." They drafted a petition which they presented to the city officials.

Two years later, Long Beach city government put an $850,000 bond issue to the vote of the people to spend $300,000 for the development and expansion of an inside passage for the Long Beach inner harbor, connecting it with Los Angeles: $500,000 for the construction of a pier, and $50,000 for building a "city hospital."

In 1921, the city adopted a Council-Manager form of government—a concept promoted nationally to professionalize the administration of local government. The council selected Charles Hewes, who had served as city manager in both Alhambra and Alameda. Hewes announced several changes concerning the City Public Health Department. The public health officer would move from his home to a city office. The department would add a public health nurse, sanitary and milk inspectors, health department clerk, statistician and veterinarian. Hewes promised that "establishment of an emergency hospital, purchase of a municipal ambulance and a rigid system of food and sanitation inspection" were planned.

A 1.9-million-dollar bond proposal by city council in 1921 funded numerous "public improvements." The council announced that a site for a general hospital had not yet been located and that until one was found, "emergency cases will be cared for in the new city hall and fire station."

The discovery of oil on Signal Hill and adjacent land would forever change the fortune of Long Beach. Not only did oil bring thousands of people to the area in search of "black gold," but the money flowed into city coffers as numerous oil wells produced an average of 25,000 barrels a day. Suddenly, Long Beach had funds to purchase land and to build a hospital. It now needed a "champion" to move plans forward.

Fillmore Condit became that champion. Condit was a descendant of John Conduit (original spelling) who came from England in the 1600s and whose ancestors included Dr. John Condit, who served in the American Revolution and in the U.S. Senate and House of Representatives for thirty years, and Silas Condit, who was a banker and member of Congress.

Condit was self-educated and began working on his father's farm and at a village store in 1867. He worked at a local sawmill but soon left to work in the meat business from 1873-1879. At the age of twenty-three, Condit invented a refrigerator door latch which brought him considerable wealth. Condit then turned to real estate on "a large scale." He was very impacted by his father's and brother's alcoholism. In 1881, he married Ida Frances Rafter. They settled in Verona, New Jersey, and raised four children and provided care for several others.

Condit immediately became involved in local affairs and donated land for a park in Verona. He was elected to the Essex County Board of Freeholders. By profession, he worked periodically in California for the Union Oil Company from 1899 to 1901. He eventually became the "resident eastern agent" for the "California Asphaltum Sales Agency" which sold asphalt for street paving. He also represented the Board of Trade Committee of California and testified before the U.S Congress concerning tariffs on asphalt imports.

In 1913, Condit was embroiled in a Tammany Hall scandal. He testified before a Grand Jury that he had been solicited by James K. McGuire for a $5,000 campaign contribution and one cent per gallon on all asphalt used by state and city contractors. The money would be required if Union Oil wanted to do business in New York. McGuire was indicted.

Condit continued being active in civic affairs and served as the president of the Board of Governors for the Hospital for Women and Children of Newark. He also dabbled in banking and steamship companies. By 1883, he was very active in the temperance movement and became an investigator, speaker and writer on the issue of the evils of saloons. He became nationally known for his anti-saloon position which found him many friends in the suffrage and white supremacy movements.

His pamphlet, *The Relation of Saloons to Insanity*, won him national acclaim and was featured as part of the publication *Guard Your Race: Address on Eugenics and Prohibition*. Condit also was publisher of the American Issue Publishing Company and Chairman of the National Saloon League. He and his wife were active in the Methodist Episcopal Church both in New Jersey and then later in Long Beach.

In 1919, Condit was so popular in the Anti-Saloon League that he was asked to be a candidate for governor of New Jersey on the Prohibition ticket. His campaign was short lived. Within months, he withdrew and supported the Republican candidate.

Condit's wife, Ida, drove to Long Beach with their adopted son, Donald. Ida informed Fillmore that Long Beach was where the family would live. She told reporters: "My husband is going to devote the remainder of his life, as a private citizen, to humanity."

It didn't take too long before Fillmore Condit became active in Long Beach politics. In 1921, he was elected to the First Council District and immediately selected by his colleagues as vice-mayor. Condit took on the challenge of championing a hospital at a time of political turmoil caused by the growing influence of the Ku Klux Klan in Long Beach.

In 1922, Condit supported the recall of recently appointed city manager, Charles Hewes. Hewes had fired the police chief who had arrested two former police chiefs for disrupting a political rally. Both were allegedly members of the KKK, which had a strong presence in Long Beach.

Condit's work for Union Oil continued and in 1922, he helped establish the Union Oil Associates, a holding company whose purpose was to keep foreign investment out of California oil.

In January 1923, the Long Beach Community Hospital Association incorporated as non-profit headed by city councilman Fillmore Condit. Other members included: Galen Welch, John M. Forsyth, L. M. Swope, W. H. Dickey, F. A. Hastings, Dr. W. E. Daniels, Annis L. Fletcher and community activist Adelaide Tichenor. Welch was a colleague on the City Council and later was named by Pres. Coolidge as a local collector of internal revenue. Forsyth was an optometrist and president of the State Optometry Board. Swope was involved in civic affairs and later appointed to the Water Commission. Dickey was a former Civil War officer, real estate broker and oilman. Daniels was a physician and secretary of the State Eclectic Medical Association. Fletcher was hired by the city in 1916 as a visiting nurse. She became superintendent of the city welfare bureau and is credited for organizing juvenile and probation services and the first children's clinic at Seaside Hospital.

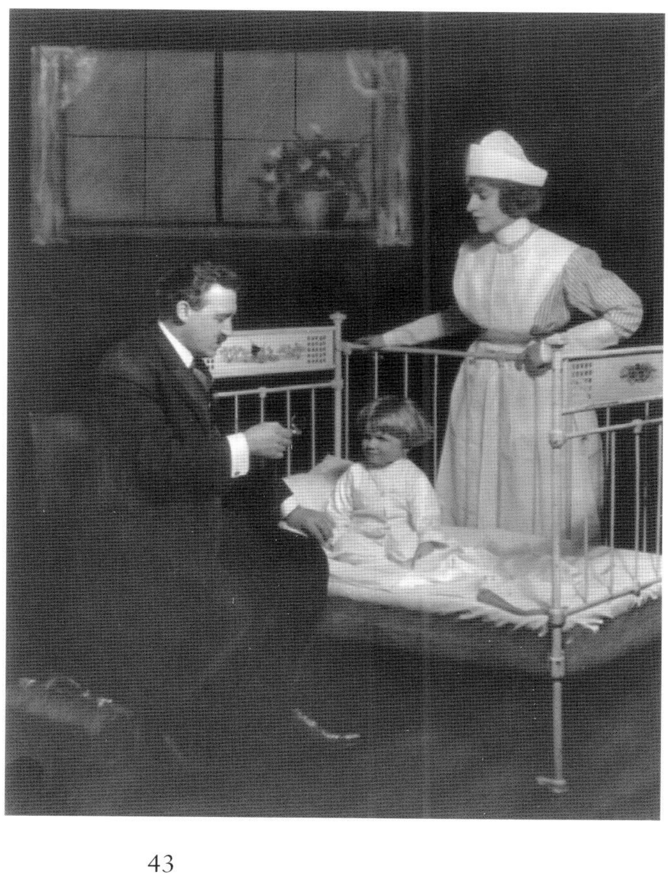

This 1919 Library of Congress photograph shows a physician making a home visit to an ill child. Physicians continued to practice out of their own homes and still relied upon elixirs composed of noxious chemicals for treatments. Hospitals were considered more and more important as advances in medicine and public health took place.

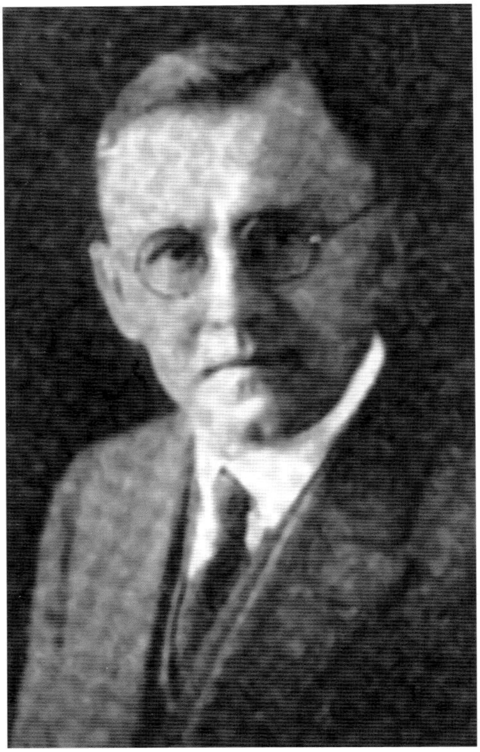

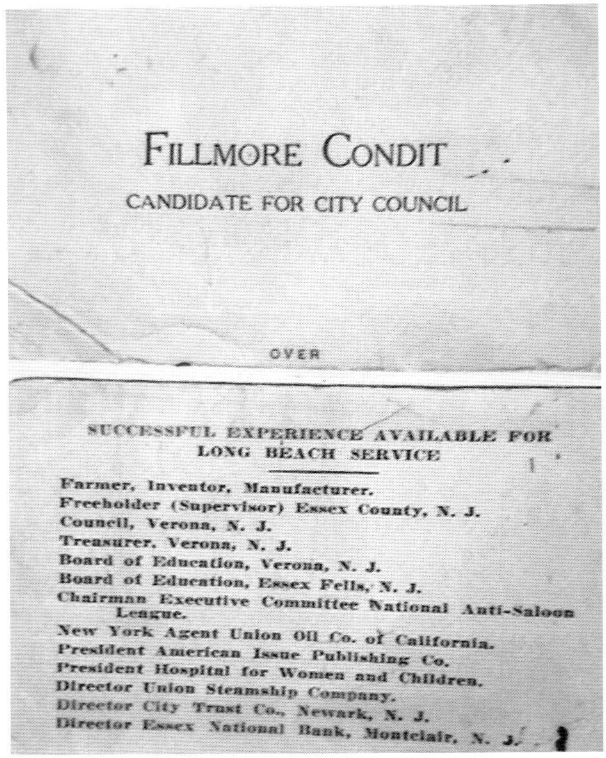

FILLMORE CONDIT

CANDIDATE FOR CITY COUNCIL

OVER

SUCCESSFUL EXPERIENCE AVAILABLE FOR LONG BEACH SERVICE

Farmer, Inventor, Manufacturer.
Freeholder (Supervisor) Essex County, N. J.
Council, Verona, N. J.
Treasurer, Verona, N. J.
Board of Education, Verona, N. J.
Board of Education, Essex Fells, N. J.
Chairman Executive Committee National Anti-Saloon League.
New York Agent Union Oil Co. of California.
President American Issue Publishing Co.
President Hospital for Women and Children.
Director Union Steamship Company.
Director City Trust Co., Newark, N. J.
Director Essex National Bank, Montclair, N. J.

Above left: In 1921, the City Council hired its first city manager, Charles Hewes. He was vice-president of the City Managers Association and considered extremely qualified. Hewes was quoted in a 1922 newspaper that in his new job he had two battles: The Southern Pacific Railroad "which insists running its freight train right down the main thoroughfare" and the many who had been political leaders in other communities before they moved to Long Beach. Hewes added that they "immediately assume the reins of government in our community and (are) the cause of no end of trouble." Hewes began reforming Long Beach city government by cutting jobs and adjusting high wages.

Above right: Fillmore Condit was a candidate for governor of New Jersey in 1919. His wife took an auto trip to Long Beach and announced that was where they were re-settling. Condit was elected in 1921 with 4,561 votes to represent the First Council District. He became part of the City Council that hired Hewes as its first city manager and quickly took on the cause of getting a "city hospital." (*HSLB*)

214,758. DOOR-FASTENERS. Fillmore Condit, Newark, N. J. Filed Nov. 16, 1878.

To all whom it may concern:

Be it known that I, FILLMORE CONDIT, of Newark, in the county of Essex and State of New Jersey, have invented a new and useful Improvement in Ice-Box-Door Fasteners, which improvement is fully described in the following specification.

My invention consists in an improved fastener for the doors of ice-boxes; and consists in the application of a wedge to the face of the door near the casing, and in pivoting a lever to a strong bolt in the door-frame, so that it may be rotated to press upon the wedge, at pleasure, or moved away from the wedge, to permit the opening of the door. As the door is more apt to stick in its casing when pressed into the same so firmly, I combine with the wedge a handle to open the door when desired.

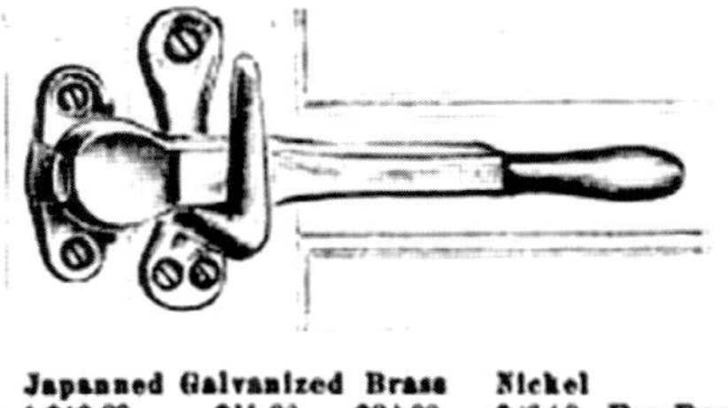

Condit was passionate about self-learning. At twenty-three, while working in meat processing, he invented a refrigerator door latch (as this patent filing indicates). The "refrigerator door fastener" invention brought him considerable wealth as it sold over a million by 1899. Condit used that money to buy real estate. (*U.S. PATENT OFFICE*)

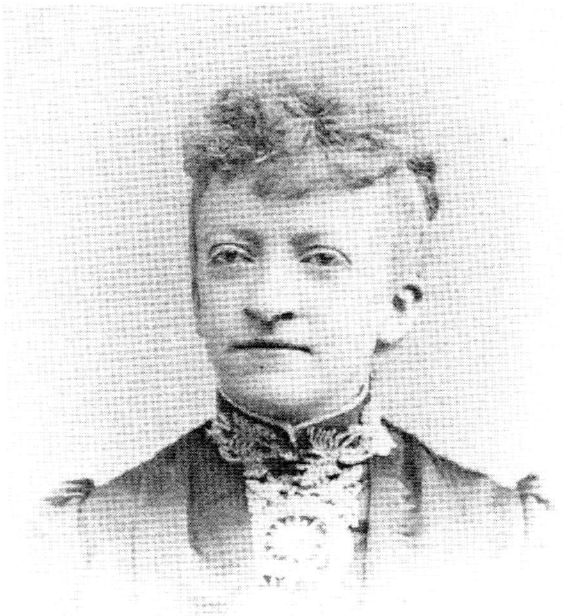

In 1881, Condit married Ida Frances Rafter. They settled in Verona, New Jersey, and raised four children. She too became successful in real estate development and joined Fillmore in many philanthropic projects. Ida served as manager of the Hospital for Women and Children in Newark and worked to find homes for destitute children. She and Fillmore adopted a child, Donald. Ida was also active in the suffrage and temperance movements. By 1921, Ida fell ill and died on April 27, 1921.

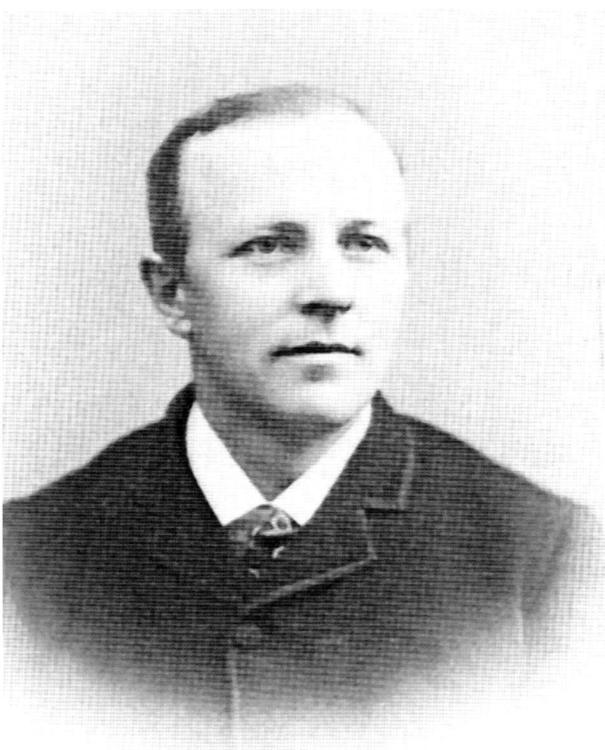

Fillmore Condit was a generous man and utilized his wealth in real estate for numerous, including donating a small park to the residents of Verona, where he served on the Board of Freeholders of Essex County. He volunteered as the president of the Board of Governors for the Hospital for Women and Children of Newark. The twenty-eight-bed hospital was established in 1882 and offered medical and surgical aid and nursing to "the women and children who are sick and disabled, suffering from acute, curable and non-contagious diseases." (*CHLBF*)

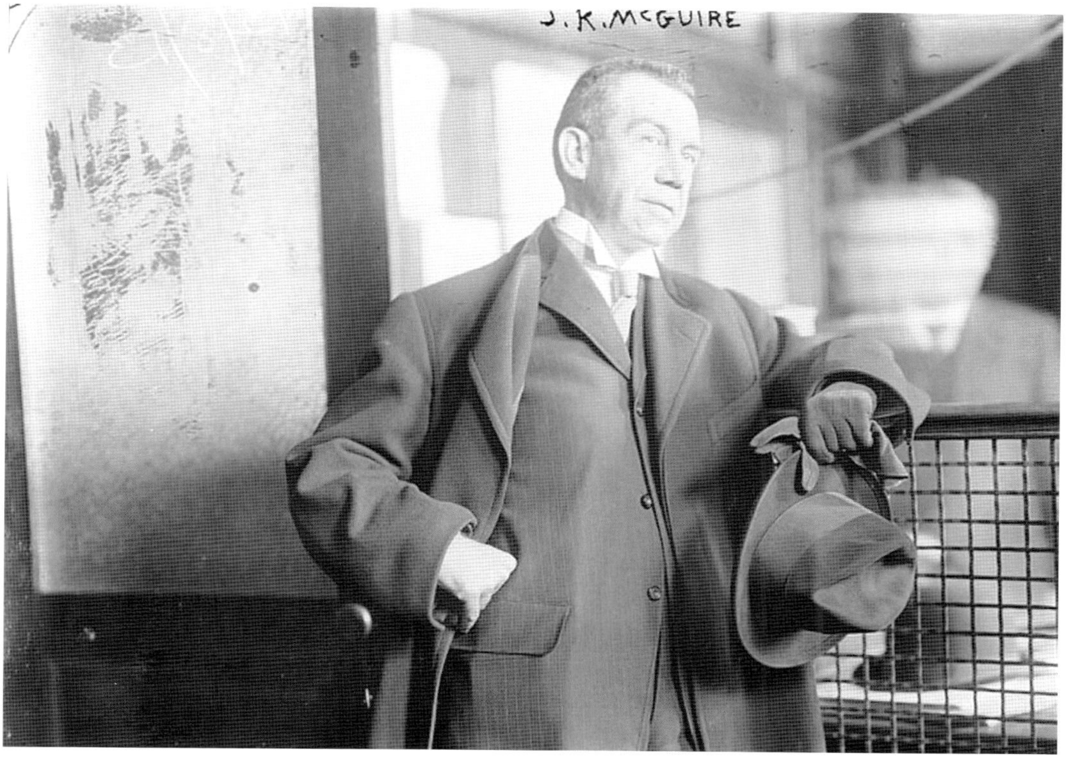

Above: In 1913, Condit testified before a Grand Jury that he had been solicited by James K. McGuire for a $5,000 campaign contribution and one-cent per gallon on all asphalt used by state and city contractors. The money would be required if Union Oil wanted sell oil-based asphalt in New York. McGuire (pictured) was the former mayor of Syracuse and a leader in the Democratic Party and the center of the Tammany Hall scandal. McGuire claimed he was being framed by the oil companies because he would not take their sides in the "natural asphalt versus oil asphalt" controversy. McGuire's brother, George, told the Grand Jury that his brother solicited the $5,000 because of his "physical and mental condition." James McGuire was indicted. (*LOC*)

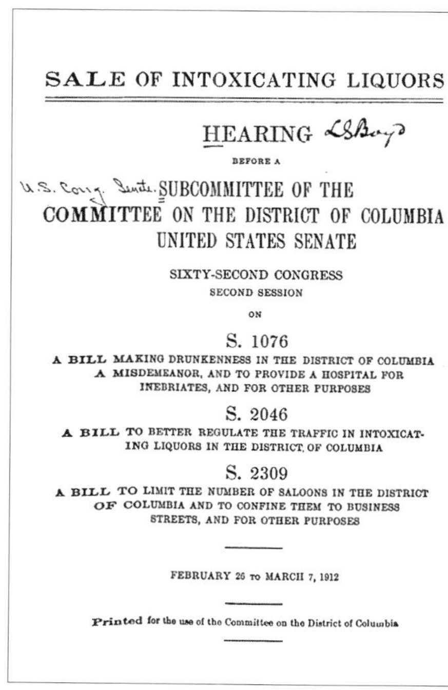

SALE OF INTOXICATING LIQUORS

HEARING

BEFORE A

SUBCOMMITTEE OF THE COMMITTEE ON THE DISTRICT OF COLUMBIA UNITED STATES SENATE

SIXTY-SECOND CONGRESS
SECOND SESSION

ON

S. 1076

A BILL MAKING DRUNKENNESS IN THE DISTRICT OF COLUMBIA A MISDEMEANOR, AND TO PROVIDE A HOSPITAL FOR INEBRIATES, AND FOR OTHER PURPOSES

S. 2046

A BILL TO BETTER REGULATE THE TRAFFIC IN INTOXICATING LIQUORS IN THE DISTRICT OF COLUMBIA

S. 2309

A BILL TO LIMIT THE NUMBER OF SALOONS IN THE DISTRICT OF COLUMBIA AND TO CONFINE THEM TO BUSINESS STREETS, AND FOR OTHER PURPOSES

FEBRUARY 26 TO MARCH 7, 1912

Printed for the use of the Committee on the District of Columbia

Right: Condit volunteered to speak and to write on the problems caused by alcohol. His pamphlet, *The Relation of Saloons to Insanity*, won national acclaim. In 1912, his pamphlet was entered into the official record of the U.S. Senate, which was proposing legislation to enforce prohibition. (*LOC*)

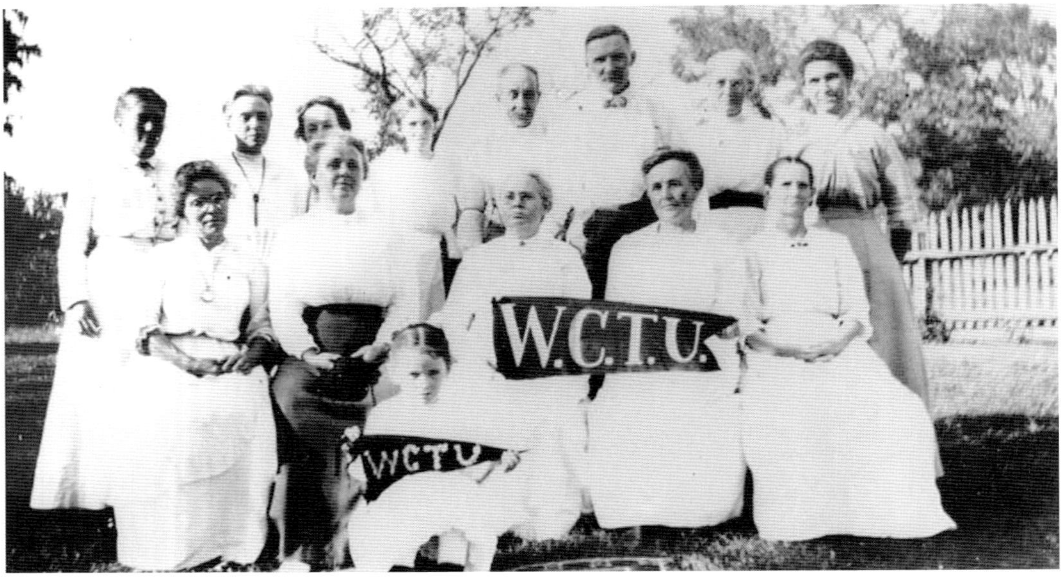

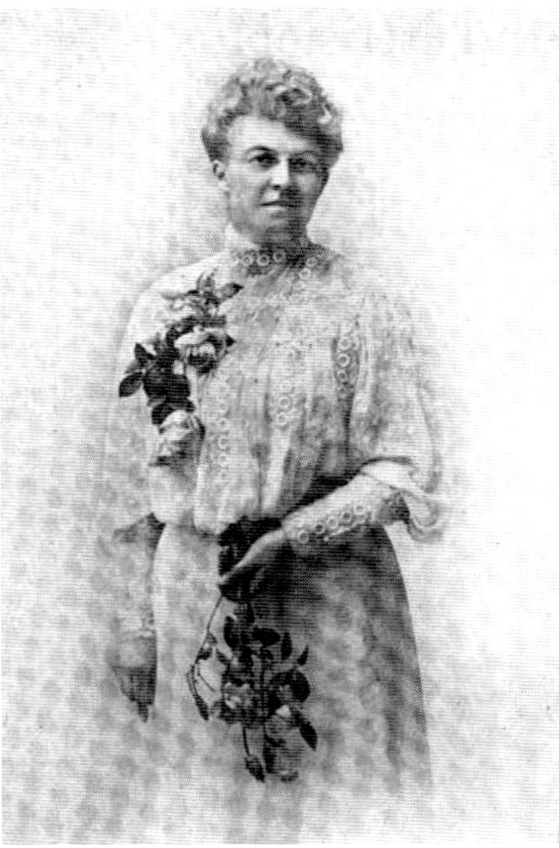

Above: In 1872, the Women's Christian Temperance Union (WCTU) was formed nationally and embraced the need to support both temperance and women's suffrage. Condit and his wife were supporters of the suffragists and were passionate about temperance. A local chapter of WCTU was active in Long Beach. (*LBPL*)

Left: Long Beach resident, Marie C. Brehm, changed her legal name to S. Marie C. Brehm—the "S" standing for suffragist. Brehm lectured on the Methodist Chautauqua circuit on both feminism and prohibition. She served as a local leader in the W.C.T.U. When Condit began championing a "people's hospital," Brehm contributed small amounts of money to the hospital and joined its board. Brehm was so influential that a 1923 news article claims she was paid a "large portion of $107,605" from water and electricity companies for her efforts to persuade women voters to vote against the "Water and Power Act." The initiative would have mandated cheaper water and power for communities.

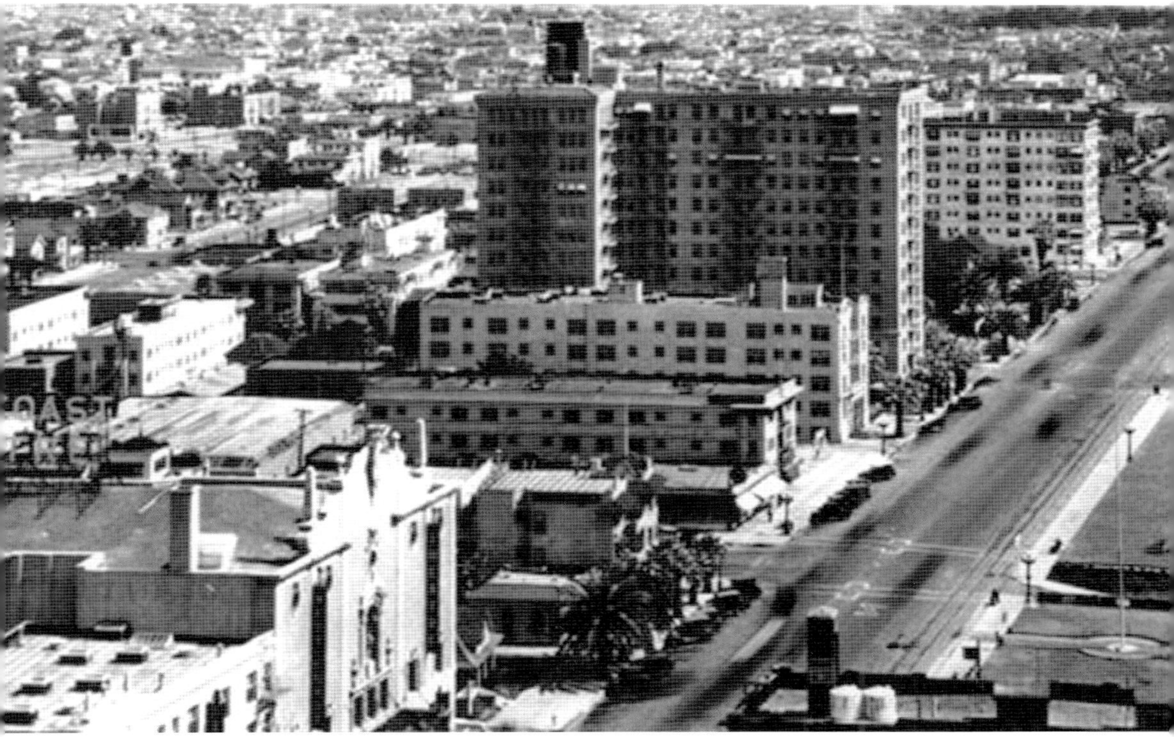

Brehm was very active locally and was appointed to the Long Beach City Planning Commission. Months later she resigned and claimed in 1923 "there was no necessity for such a commission, as practically all its recommendations are ignored by the city council." She was referring to the fact that Council ignored the Commission's opposition to increasing building heights on Ocean Boulevard (shown in 1920 photograph), "thus cutting the rest of the city from a view of the sea." (*USCA*)

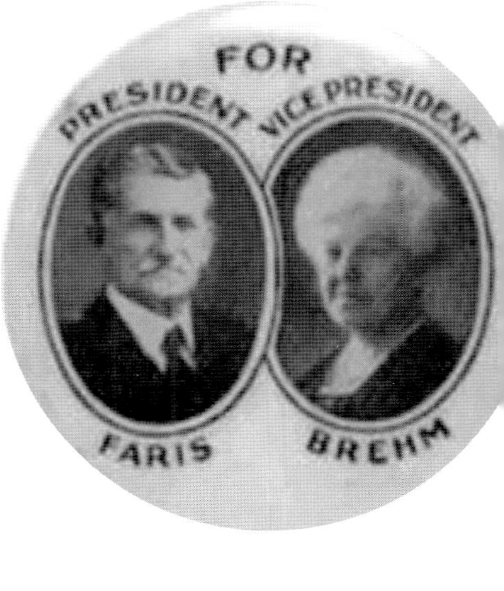

In 1920, Marie Brehm of Long Beach became the first woman in the history of national politics to be elected chair of a major convention. Brehm was nominated by the Prohibition Party as its candidate for vice-president of the U.S. in 1924. She was one of eleven on the Council of One Hundred who framed the Volstead Act and held out for the substitution of the word "alcoholic" for "intoxicating" when referring to liquor that would be barred. She was concerned that "medicinal" and "sacramental" liquids containing alcohol would still flow. While attending the "Pageant of Roses" in Pasadena in 1926, the grand stand collapsed. Brehm suffered head wounds and died shortly after. She loved the new community hospital and left it $1,000 in her will. A "temperance room" was dedicated in her honor in the early Long Beach Community Hospital. (*LOC*)

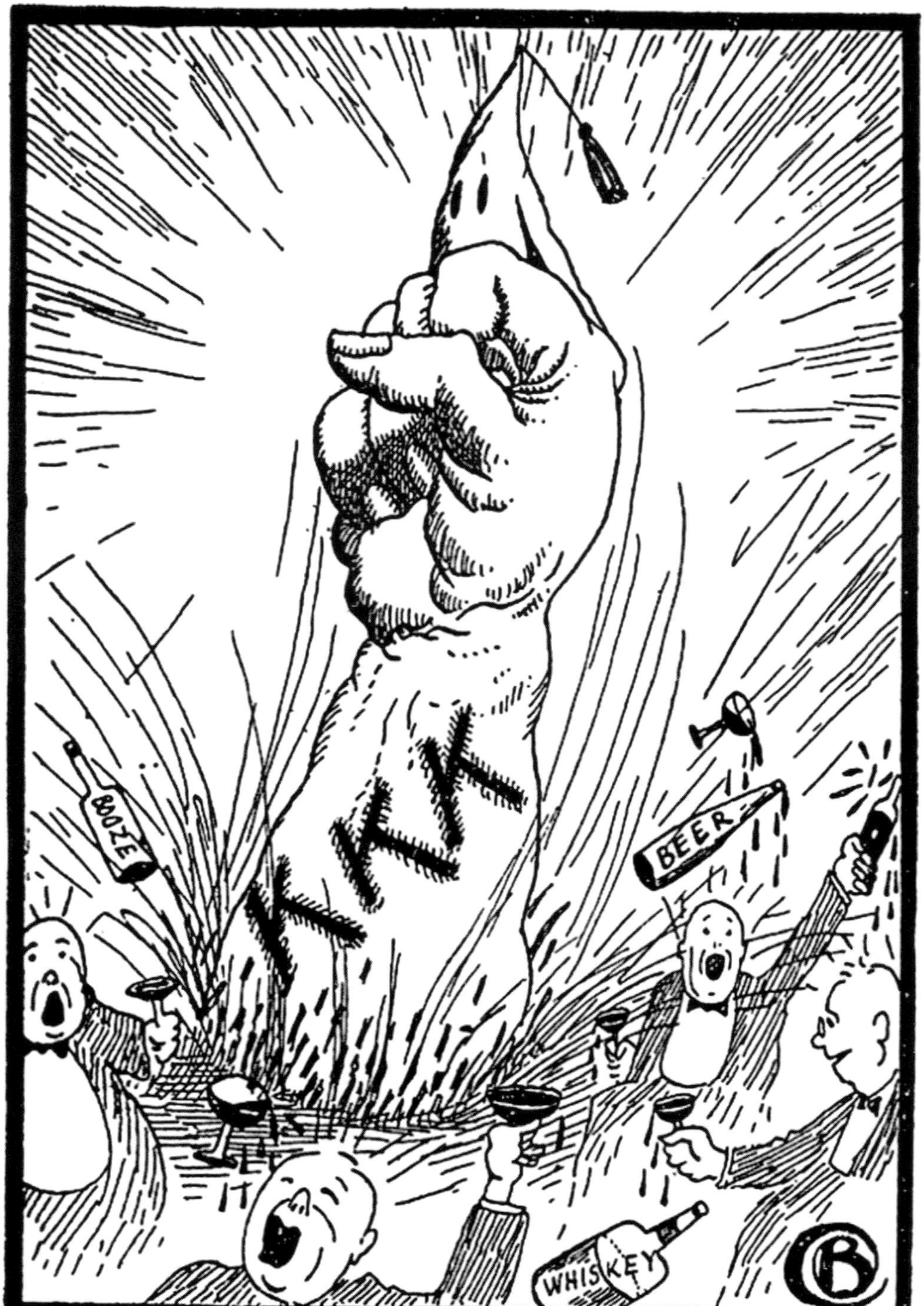
KKK
BOOZE
BEER
WHISKEY

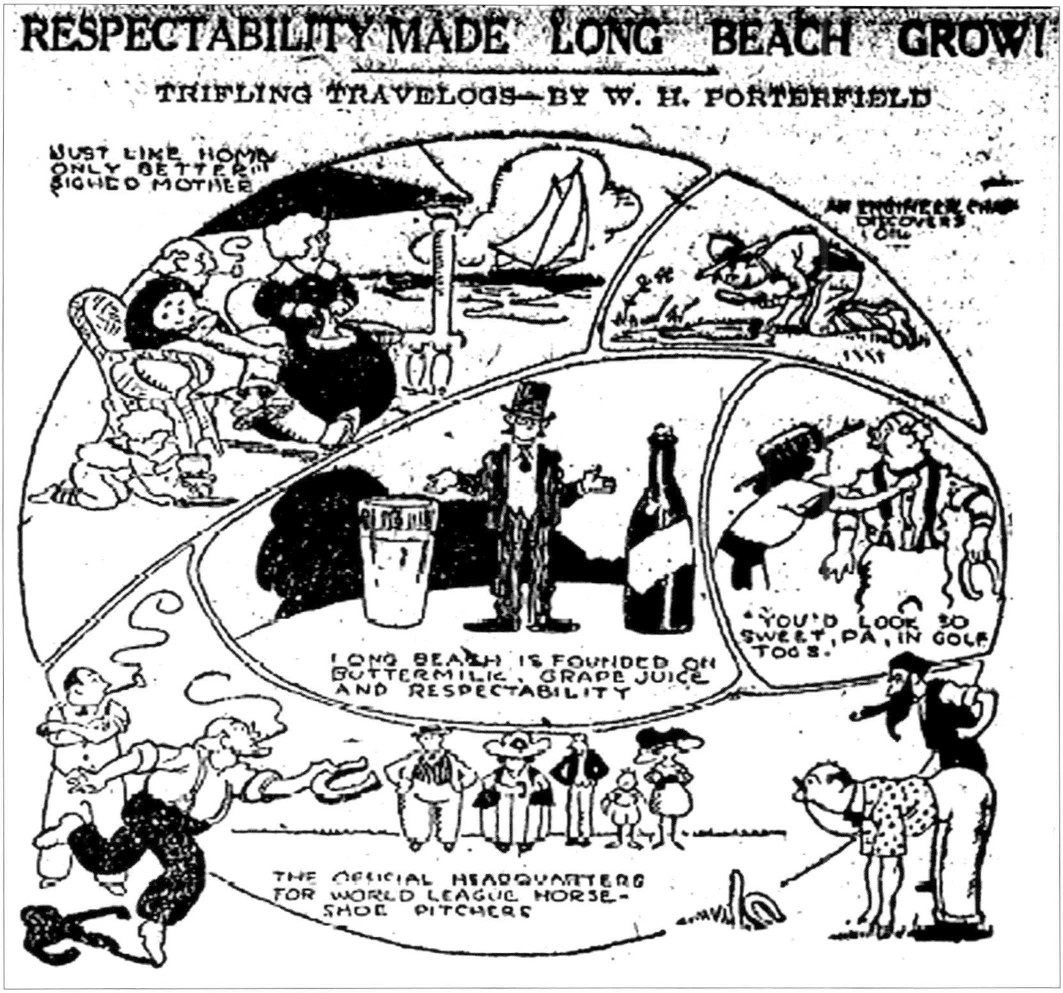
RESPECTABILITY MADE LONG BEACH GROW!
TRIFLING TRAVELOGS—BY W. H. PORTERFIELD
JUST LIKE HOME ONLY BETTER!" SIGHED MOTHER
LONG BEACH IS FOUNDED ON BUTTERMILK, GRAPE JUICE AND RESPECTABILITY
"YOU'D LOOK SO SWEET, PA, IN GOLF TOGS."
THE OFFICIAL HEADQUARTERS FOR WORLD LEAGUE HORSE-SHOE PITCHERS

From its first incorporation in 1888, Long Beach was a "dry" city. The anti-prohibition supporters moved to un-incorporate Long Beach in 1896 to make it county property and thus free to sell liquor. The city reincorporated in 1897 and limited the sale of alcohol to those who had a physician order. Many news articles attributed the growth of Long Beach to the fact that it was "saloon-less," as pictured in the 1922 *Freeport Journal*, Freeport, Illinois.

Opposite: Many in the temperance and suffragist movements were also advocates of white supremacy. Fillmore Condit's writings on the link of saloons with insanity were also featured as part of the publication *Guard Your Race: Address on Eugenics and Prohibition*. In the early 1920s, the Knights of the Ku Klux Klan were very popular in some regions of the country, including Long Beach. The KKK "enforced" prohibition efforts in several communities. Thousands of KKK gathered at the Long Beach auditorium to hear local WCTU official, Marie Brehm, speak in 1923 and then paraded down Ocean Boulevard. (*LOC*)

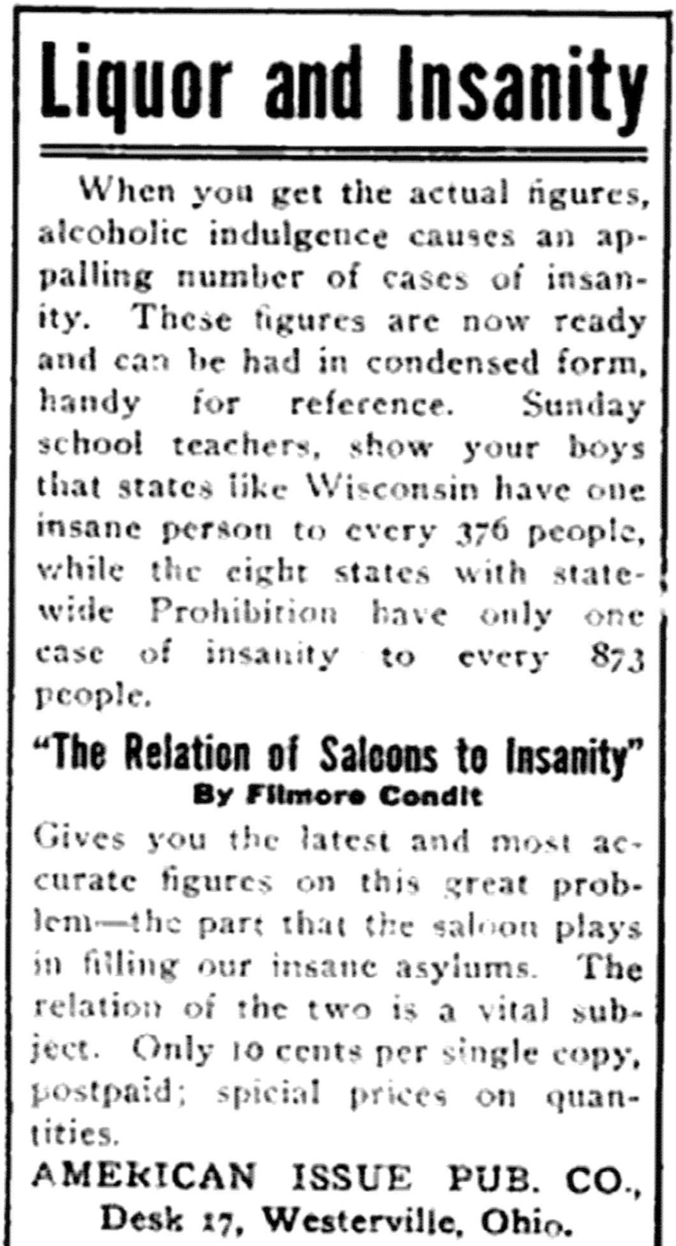

Liquor and Insanity

When you get the actual figures, alcoholic indulgence causes an appalling number of cases of insanity. These figures are now ready and can be had in condensed form, handy for reference. Sunday school teachers, show your boys that states like Wisconsin have one insane person to every 376 people, while the eight states with statewide Prohibition have only one case of insanity to every 873 people.

"The Relation of Saloons to Insanity"
By Filmore Condit

Gives you the latest and most accurate figures on this great problem—the part that the saloon plays in filling our insane asylums. The relation of the two is a vital subject. Only 10 cents per single copy, postpaid; spicial prices on quantities.

AMERICAN ISSUE PUB. CO.,
Desk 17, Westerville, Ohio.

Fillmore Condit was very active in the Methodist Episcopal Church both in New Jersey and then later in Long Beach. He served as the chairman of the American Issue Publishing Company, the holding company of the Anti-Saloon League. AIP printed and disseminated information on the "evils of saloons." Condit also was elected chairman of the National Executive Committee of the Anti-Saloon League. (*LOC*)

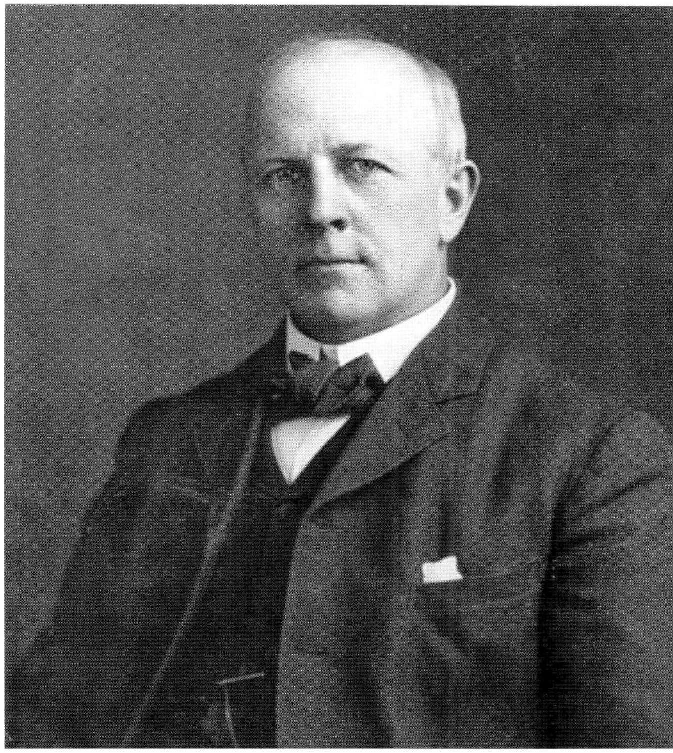

Right: It didn't take long before Fillmore Condit became active in Long Beach politics. His wife died in April, and in June 1921, he was elected to the First Council District, defeating Dr. Lewis Crutcher and Mary Tanner. Condit was immediately selected as vice-mayor by his colleagues. (*CHLBF*)

Below: One of Condit's first initiatives was to encourage the city to close the Pike and Silver Spray pier "cider stands" because of a wave of public intoxication. An investigation found that the source of the alcohol was a local drug store at Broadway and American where the druggist would mix a concoction for $3.75.

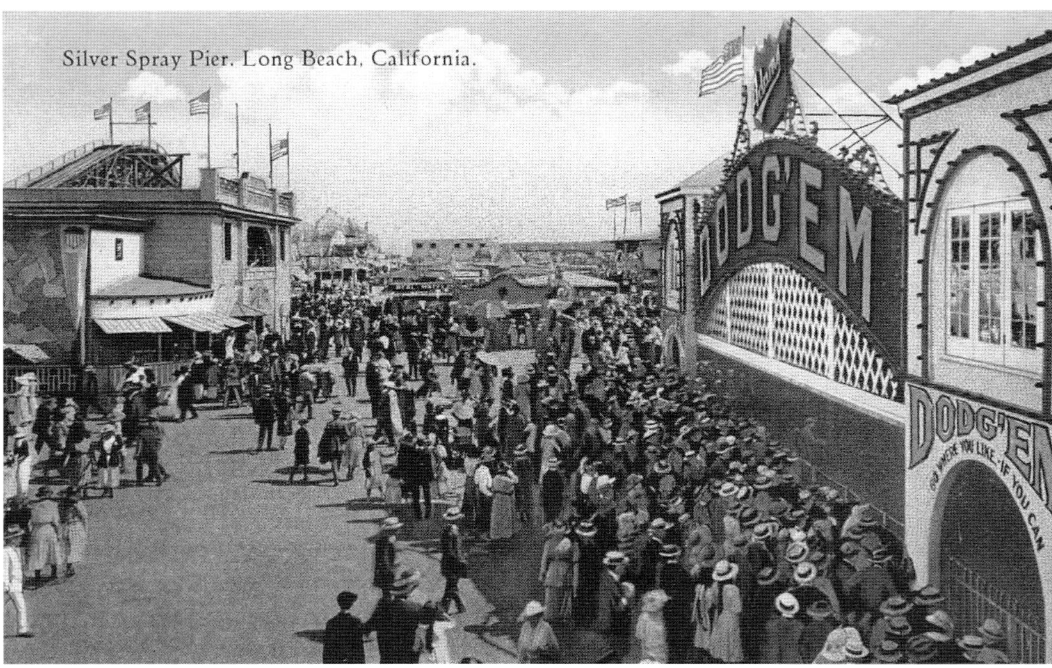

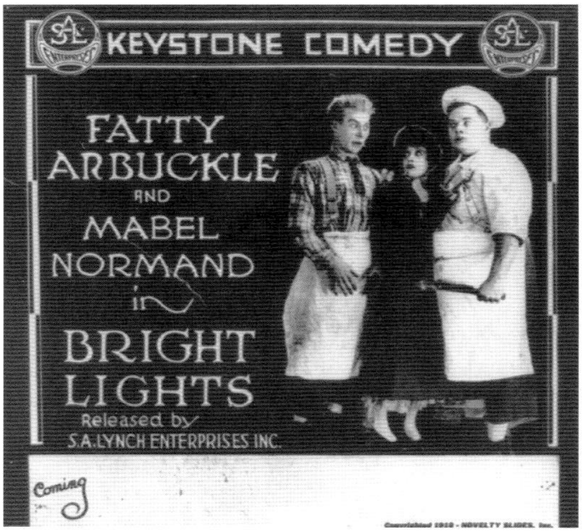

In 1924, the *Los Angeles Times* reported that Condit supported the Women of the KKK who came to City Council and proposed keeping movie actor Fatty Arbuckle from appearing on local stages. Arbuckle had been acquitted of murdering his girlfriend only to be confronted by Councilman Condit, who made a motion to prevent Arbuckle from making public appearances in Long Beach because of his "drunkenness." Condit's motion was tabled, and Arbuckle continued to perform in Long Beach. (*LOC*)

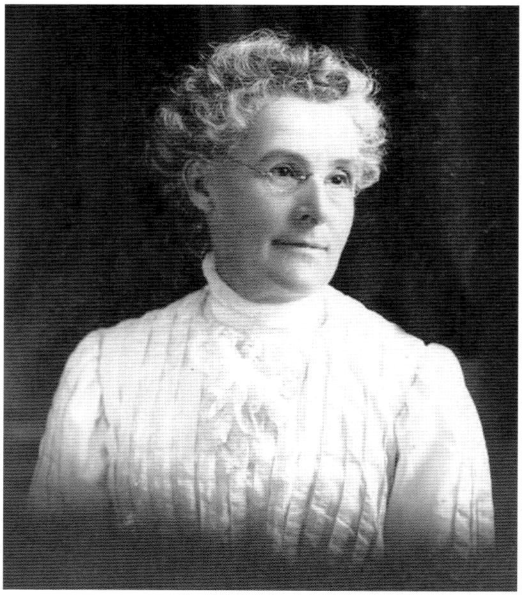

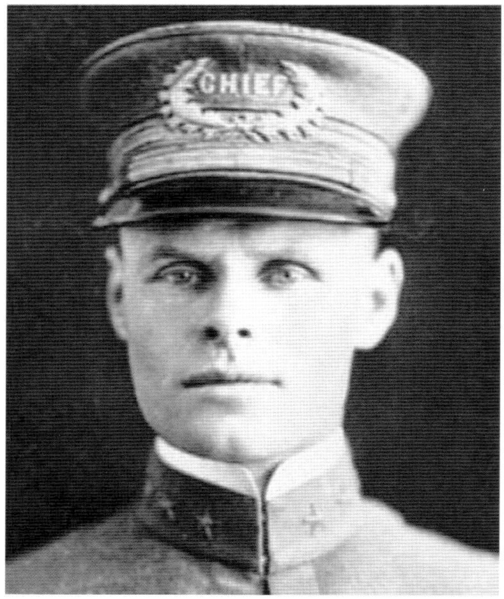

Above left: Adelaide Tichenor, a native of Kansas, came to Long Beach in 1894. A generous philanthropist, Tichenor donated land for the Long Beach Day Nursery and gave considerable money to the Community Hospital.

Above right: The KKK grew in popularity in the 1920s in Long Beach. City Manager Hewes was given a list of more than 180 city employees who might be members of the Ku Klux Klan. Hewes announced his policy that KKK membership would be forbidden. Chief of Police Ben McClendon issued "Special Order 17" which made clear that no member of the police department could be a member of the KKK. McClendon arrested two former police chiefs (Charles Cole and James Butterfield [pictured]) for disturbing a political rally. Hewes fired McClendon and then Hewes was recalled by voters in a special election just weeks later.

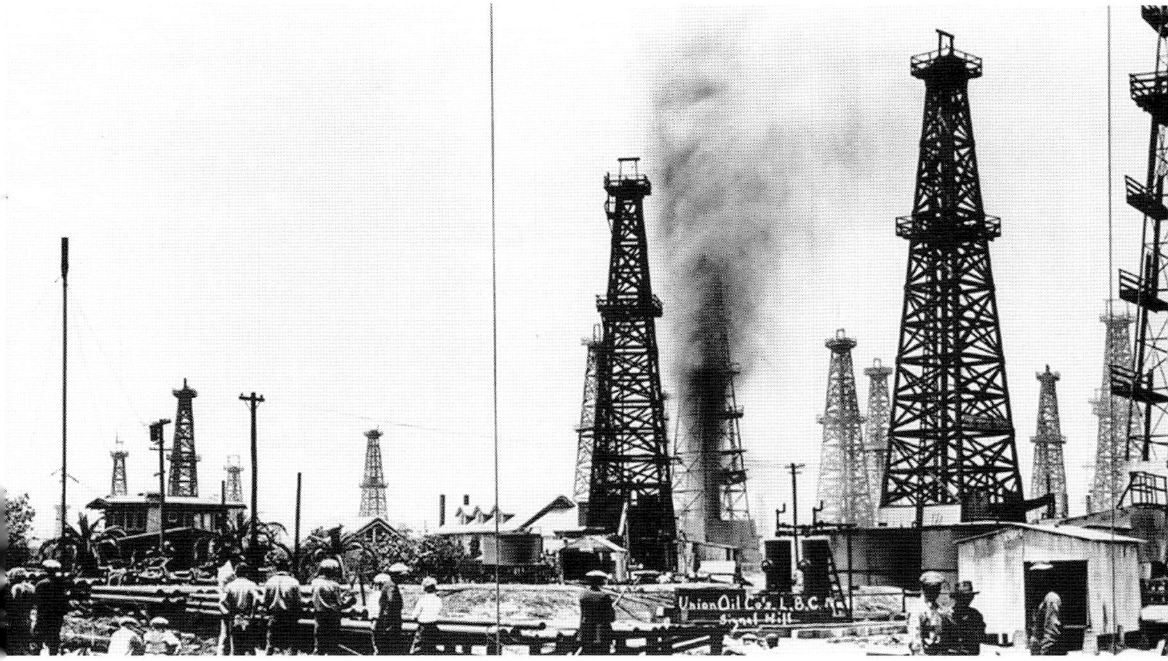

Above: When the Alamitos #1 drilling site hit oil, Long Beach became wealthy overnight. Within months, oil flowed from thousands of derricks at a rate of 1,500 barrels a day at each site. City Manager Hewes proclaimed, before he was recalled, that the oil would bring the city $300,000 which could be used for major civic improvements such as an "emergency hospital." (*USGS*)

Right: Almost every inch of Long Beach and Signal Hill were covered with oil derricks or other drilling devices after oil was discovered. The city selected an 8-acre site for the new community hospital, which was being drilled by W. R. Ramsey (pictured) of Oklahoma, who had rights to drill for oil on 120 acres. The city asked Ramsey to give back his oil drilling lease. Ramsey later became a founder of Conoco Oil Company. To ensure that no one else could drill near the hospital site, Condit pushed state legislation that prohibited oil drilling within 500 feet of hospitals. (*LOC*)

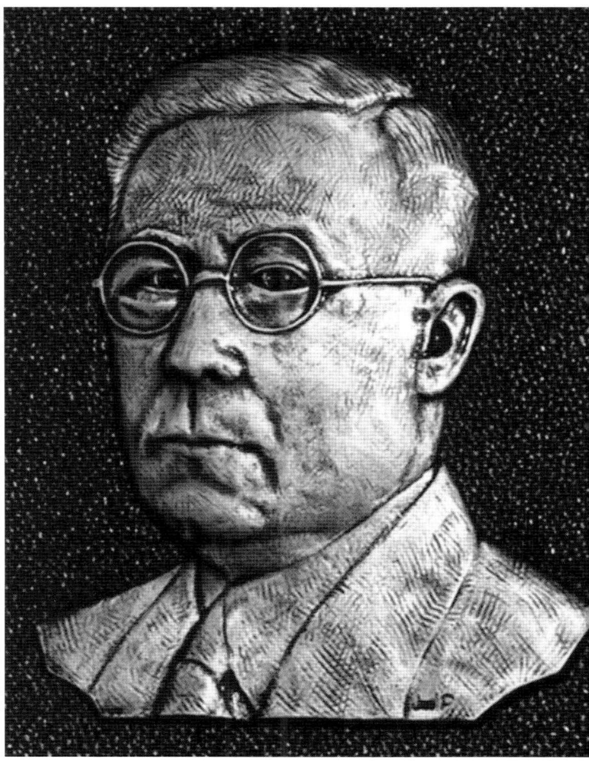

6

Community Hospital: (1924-?)

> I think there is no better philanthropy than doing for the sick in one's own city. When I was in social work in Long Beach, we had no place but the county hospital to send our sick people to, so far away that their relatives could not visit them often, and frequently the county hospital was too crowded to give them proper care.
>
> A note from Fanny Bixby Spencer to Long Beach Community Hospital

Voters approved $100,000 in bonds in 1922 to purchase land and to hire an architect to design the new hospital. Arguments ensued about the location and the design. The 8-acre site of "Oil No. 5 Reservoir" near Farm Lot No. 39, Alamitos Tract at Termino Avenue and State Street (Pacific Coast Highway) was selected. Once Oklahoma oilman W. R. Ramsey willingly relinquished his drilling lease on the site, the council authorized an additional $100,000 for construction.

Mayor Fillmore Condit, chairman of the hospital committee, and several others, personally pledged to donate additional money. Over his lifetime, Condit generously gave more than $150,000 for the hospital, sometimes contributing to meet payroll.

Long Beach architect, Hugh R. Davies, was selected to design the hospital. He personally donated $3,000 to the hospital association. His "unit plan" hospital utilized the modern "wing" concept. The administration office was placed in the front and the different "units" on the sides with a courtyard. Modern hospitals no longer looked like sanitariums. The "modern" hospital had private suites and multi-patient wards.

The public was asked to donate furnishings and money when the hospital was completed. More than 1,300 individuals, churches, banks and civic associations, including Long Beach Ku Klux Klan #1 of the Realm of California, raised the money needed to open the "people's hospital" that was neither Catholic or private. Condit told reporters in 1932 that the city spent one-half million to build Community and to fight off oil speculators who filled the area with drilling sites.

Months before the opening of Community Hospital, the Executive Board of the hospital voted to exclude osteopaths, chiropractors and "members from other schools" from controlling or practicing at the hospital. The vote reflected the ongoing battle between medical doctors and other practitioners and the growing power of the American Medical

Association. The City Council affirmed the vote of the hospital and was sued by osteopaths on the basis that the city owned the property and had funded most of the construction and could not restrict who could practice medicine. A settlement was reached years later.

Long Beach Community Hospital Association Board member, Adelaide Tichenor, was affectionately referred to as the "mother of Long Beach clubs" for founding the Ebell Club, the City Club and many other civic and women's organizations. She was instrumental in persuading Andrew Carnegie to donate $30,000 for construction of a new library. Tichenor died in 1924 before the hospital opened. She left $200,000 in her will for construction of a hospital for "crippled children." The Adelaide Tichenor Orthopedic Clinic opened in 1926 in the Community Hospital. In 1938, it opened a separate facility adjacent to the hospital and continues to serve the community.

Community Hospital opened on July 15,1924, and within twelve months had treated more than 1,800 patients. The stated purpose of the city financing a community hospital was to provide "hospital care for cost" for Long Beach residents or "service without profit" as Condit told the press. Miss Blanche Starr, R.N., was appointed the hospital's first administrator.

Community Hospital established "public welfare clinics" to take care of the growing number of patients without money. Condit lobbied the county of Los Angeles to build a hospital in Long Beach to take the poorest of patients.

In 1930, the city constructed the Alamitos Traffic Circle in anticipation of the traffic the 1932 Olympics might bring to the newly constructed Marine Stadium. The "roundabout" was located immediately below Community Hospital. Consequently, countless victims of traffic accidents have been taken there over the years.

The March 10, 1933, a 6.7-magnitude Long Beach earthquake devastated most of the city's school buildings and severely damaged Seaside and St. Mary's Hospital. The first night, 125 were treated and ninety were hospitalized. Over the next ten days, the staff of Community would treat 500 injured. The hospital sustained little damage.

By 1939, the hospital opened the area's first "Tumor and Cancer Diagnostic Clinic." The same year, Fillmore Condit died at Community Hospital at age eighty-three. He is buried with his first wife in Caldwell, New Jersey.

Months after Condit's death, local press featured a front-page scathing rebuke of Community Hospital, claiming the city was getting nothing in return for the money the city had given, and that Community was not providing "low cost care" as intended. The article noted that the city was only receiving "$12 over the course of a 10-year lease." Criticism died down during WWII.

A new wing opened, increasing patient beds to 150. In 1949, 8,400 patients were cared for, and 1,328 babies born. Throughout the 1950s, the hospital continued to expand, adding the "Howard Hatfield Memorial Wing" in memory of the hospital's former administrator. The wing offered a scenic view of Lakewood and Los Altos areas through wide-glass windows. Hospital rates ranged from $12 a day for a ward room to $17 for a private room. Women were kept in the hospital a week to twelve days after delivering a baby, at a rate of $126.50 for a ward and $141.00 for private rooms. Nursery charges were $2.50 a day and $3.50 for "preemies." By 1956, 5,000 surgical procedures had been performed in the hospital.

Community created the first "convalescent" unit in an acute care hospital in 1958. It included a "lounge area" surrounded by glass to provide restful views. In 1959, a

$2.5-million, six-story east wing doubled bed capacity to 300. The funds came from 10 million dollars in bonds approved by voters in 1956. The six-story expansion included a larger maternity wing located on the fourth floor. The unit reflected the post-war "baby boom" and included an anesthesia recovery room, isolation nursery and five eight-bassinet nurseries. A pediatric unit was located on the fifth floor, complete with a sun deck, two isolation rooms and a television room. To facilitate medical education, a 275-seat auditorium was built on the northern side of the facility.

In 1960, the City of Long Beach issued $10,500,000 in bonds that were used to build Memorial Hospital and to expand Community, Long Beach Osteopathic and St. Mary's. Community utilized the funds to remodel and restore the original hospital buildings. More than one-half million was spent in equipping the expansion.

The hospital continued to be leased from the City of Long Beach by the Long Beach Community Hospital Association for $10 a year. An intensive care unit was added in 1965 and a nuclear medicine department in 1967.

The 1970s brought dramatic changes to healthcare. Cost controls were put in place by insurance companies through "managed care" and revenues fell for hospitals. Community struggled to compete with the several other area hospitals and in 1976 established a foundation to assist in raising funds.

In 1980, the City of Long Beach designated the oldest part of the hospital as a "historical landmark" because of its distinctive design and significance to the city.

Community attempted to stay competitive and affiliated with Healthwest in the 1980s. Healthwest also struggled and merged with LHS to become Unihealth. A psychiatric unit and sexual assault forensic examination room were added to Community. The Harriman Jones Medical Group officially joined Community Hospital after a three-year affiliation.

The *Los Angeles Times* noted that in the late 1980s and early 1990s, Community Hospital employees contributed over $1.3 million to fund improvement projects at the hospital. Their "charity" surpassed most other Long Beach businesses.

After Healthwest sold its facilities and leases to Catholic Healthcare West in 1998, Community continued to struggle. Not five miles away, another Catholic Healthcare West hospital, St. Mary Medical Center, was a direct competitor.

Community Hospital lost more than $13 million in 1999 and Catholic Healthcare West announced the closure of Community the next year. The announcement drew an investigation by the State Attorney General and public outcry. The hospital was closed in October.

A group of residents formed "Save Our Neighborhood Hospital" and rallied to urge the City of Long Beach to allow them to operate a "new" Community Hospital: "Community Hospital of Long Beach." It opened in June 2001 with funds raised by the group and the hospital's foundation. The "new" hospital had fewer than seventy-five beds.

The city leased the property for one dollar a year and provided a "tenant improvement loan." It also billed the group for having to maintain the site after Catholic Healthcare West closed it. Community Hospital of Long Beach was to repay the City of Long Beach $2,288,579 or $184,160 per year.

The group which took over Community Hospital in 2001 had been given a staggering 23-million-dollar assessment to seismically retrofit or close the emergency room and other acute care services. By 2011, the group was unable to financially continue, and operations were taken over by Memorial Medical Care.

While Memorial Medical Care improved some infrastructure at Community, it decided early on in its lease with the city, that the state seismic retrofit requirements made it impossible to continue acute care services beyond 2019.

In 2018, Memorial Medical Care terminated its lease with the City of Long Beach and would no longer operate Community Hospital of Long Beach. It is unknown what will happen to this city-owned historic hospital.

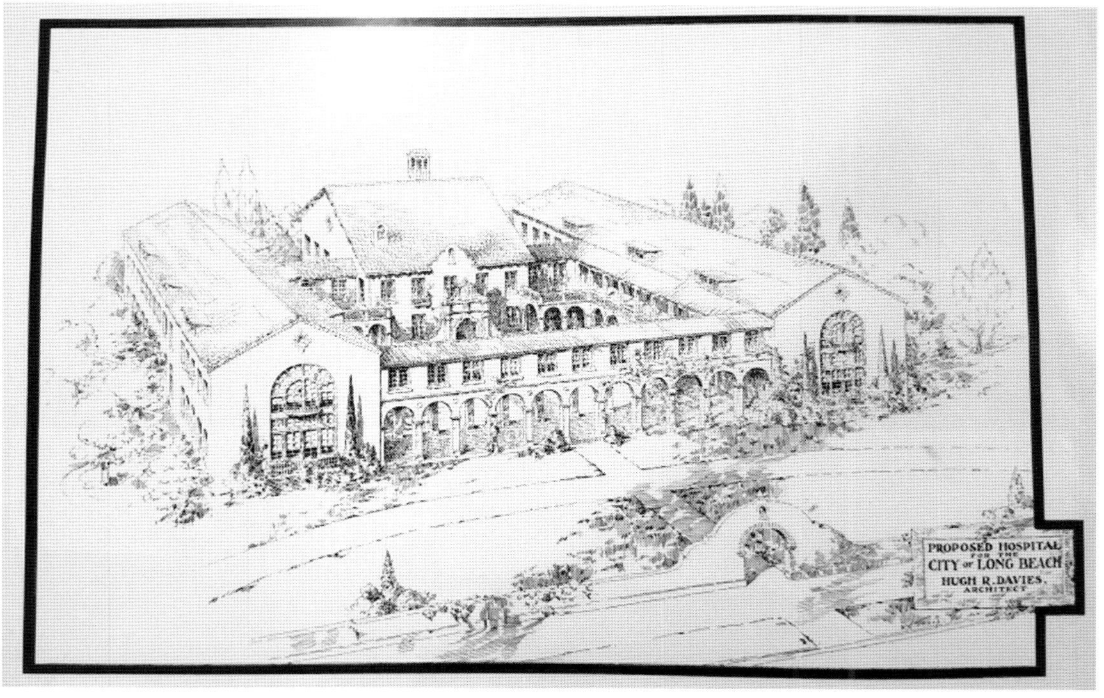
PROPOSED HOSPITAL
FOR THE
CITY OF LONG BEACH
HUGH R. DAVIES,
ARCHITECT

The Long Beach Community Hospital Association hired local architect, Hugh R. Davies, to design the hospital in a modern "unit" design which utilized the modern "wing" concept. The administration office was placed in the front and the different "units" on the sides with a courtyard. Modern hospitals no longer looked like sanitariums. The "modern" hospital had a "home atmosphere" with private suites and multi-patient wards. (*CHLBF*).

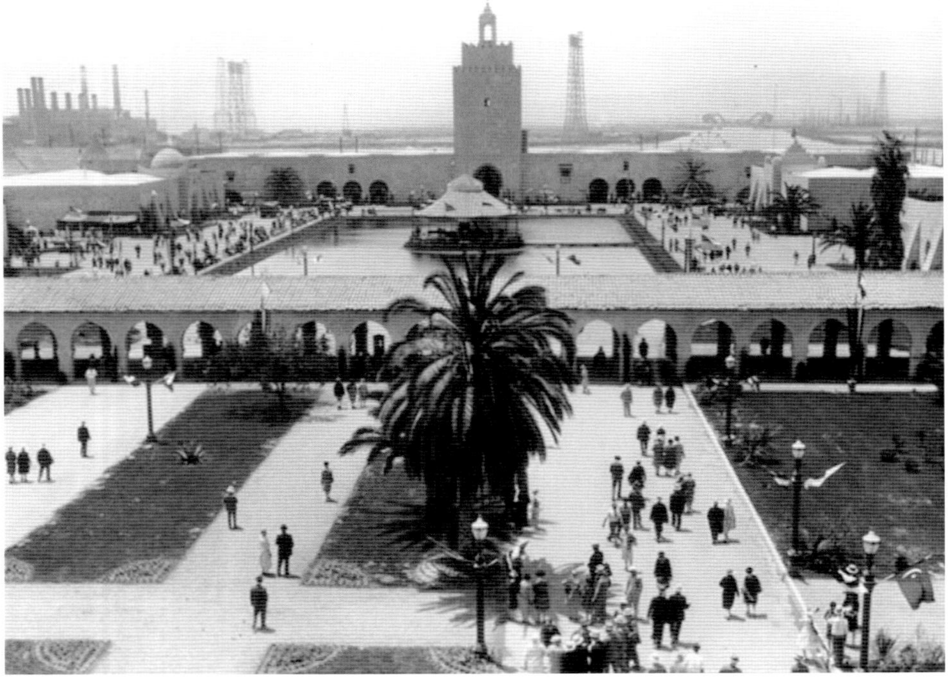

Architect Hugh R. Davies' designs were highly influenced by his travels in the Middle East and in Morocco. After designing Community Hospital, Davies designed: Pacific Southwest Exhibition buildings (pictured) (1928), the Pacific Clinic Orthopedic Hospital (1931), the Mottell Mortuary and Chapel (pictured) (1932), and an updated Long Beach Poly High School (1933).

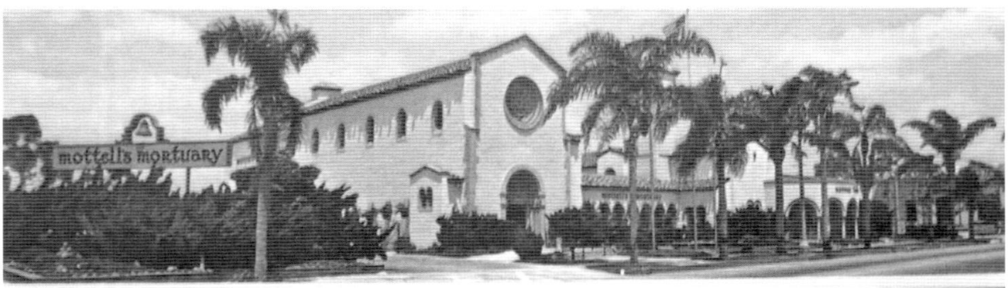

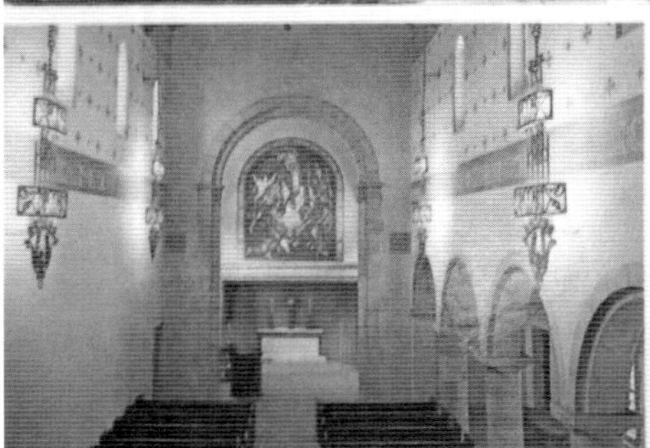

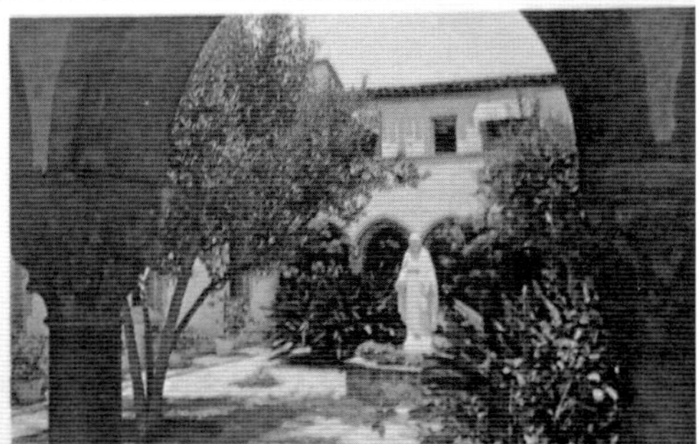

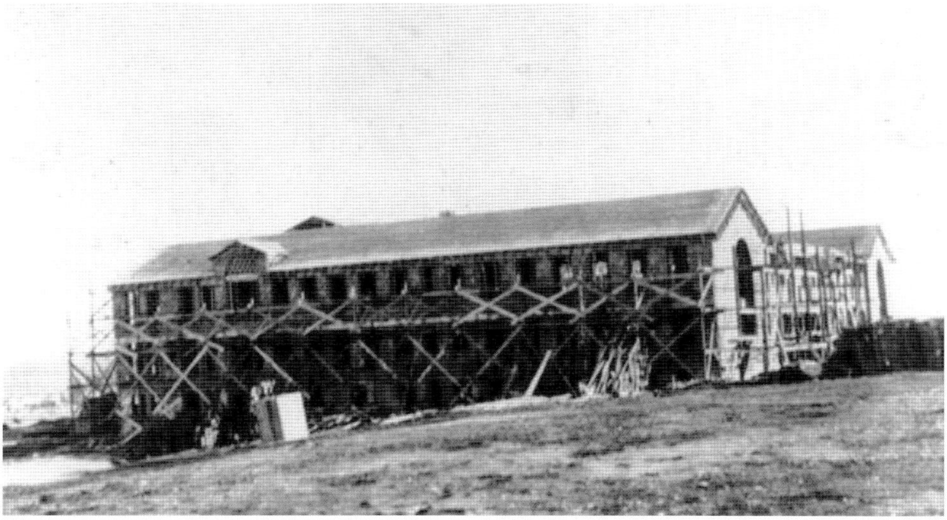

Construction of the hospital was supervised by Herbert Murphy, who, forty years later, joined the Community Hospital Association Board of Directors.

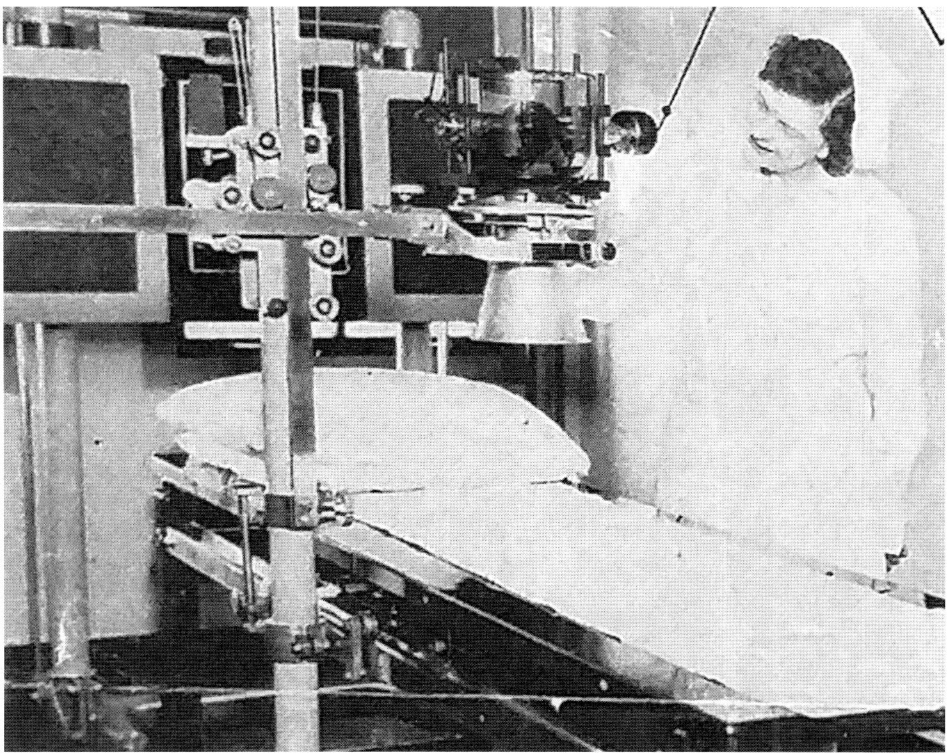

Within a few years of opening, Community Hospital purchased the latest in technology—an x-ray machine known as a "Wappler."

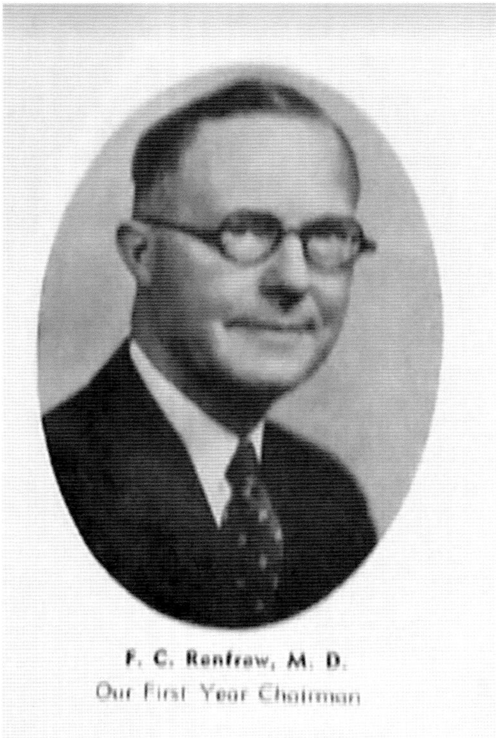

Left: Months before the opening of Community Hospital, the Executive Board of the hospital voted to exclude osteopaths, chiropractors and "members of other schools," from controlling or practicing at the hospital. Only members of the American Medical Association could be on staff. F. C. Renfrew, M.D. became the first chairman of the medical staff. (*CHLBF*)

Opposite: Long Beach Community Hospital Association Board member, Adelaide Tichenor, disclosed in 1923 that she would endow a "crippled children's" hospital in her will. She left $200,000 in her will from funds she had inherited from the sale of land when her husband, Lester died. The Adelaide Tichenor Orthopedic Clinic opened in 1926 in a room in the Community Hospital. In 1938, it opened a separate facility adjacent to the hospital, as noted in the 1938 *Journal of Physiotherapy Review.*

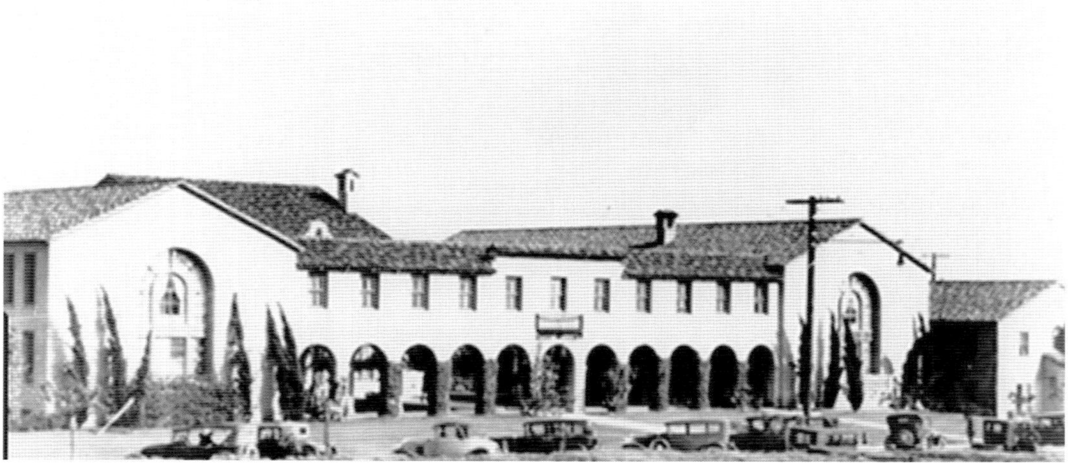

Community Hospital opened on July 15,1924, with the help of numerous financial contributions, including $500 from the Long Beach Ku Klux Klan #1 of the Realm of California. The hospital offered 100 beds: twenty-four were private suites and the remainder were multi-patient wards. There were two operating rooms and a dressing room for the 175 physicians who practiced there. During its first year, more than 1,900 patients were given care and 302 babies were born, including Fillmore Condit's granddaughter, Barbara.

The New Building for the Adelaide Tichenor Clinic in Long Beach, California

Gladdes B. Neff

The beautiful new building housing the Adelaide Tichenor Orthopedic Clinic is completed. Trustees, directors, and the staff, proud and happy, escorted some 1500 visitors through the structure on the opening day—January 29, 1938. Now the city of Long Beach at large is better acquainted with the general nature of the work the clinic is performing for the handicapped children of the community.

The Clinic was established eleven years ago through the benevolence of Mrs. Adelaide Tichenor who was impressed with the aid which a well established clinic would give the many children suffering from structural deficiencies. Accordingly, she caused to be inserted in her will the provision that has made possible this clinic for treatment of orthopedic cases.

As one approaches the building one is impressed with the beauty of exterior design. It is of a modern type of architecture with simple straight lines and is designed to provide the maximum of air and light. The building is one story in height, of cream colored stucco, erected at the corner of Wilton and Termino streets. It is placed on a spacious site which has been artistically landscaped to set off to best advantage the beauty of the structure.

As the institution enters its new building it records a total of 1650 cases having come under its treatment in eleven years. Many of these are discharged as having had the maximum amount of treatment necessary for sound citizenry.

A fine balance between the aesthetic and the practical characterizes the interior. A study of many outstanding clinics was made before this one was evolved, and the best features of many have been used.

The predominant color scheme of the interior is cream and desert tan. Entering an attractive reception room furnished in raffia with golden draperies, one is impressed with its spaciousness. To the right is the business office where patients are entered and checked out. To the left is a children's library of striking design and ornamentation. A colorful frieze around the top of this room delights the little patients with the many doings of "Little Black Sambo." This was done by a Long Beach High School girl who deserves great credit. Beyond the library is a suite of rooms for the technicians, consisting of a kitchen which is equipped with an electric refrigerator and range, a very attractive lounging room

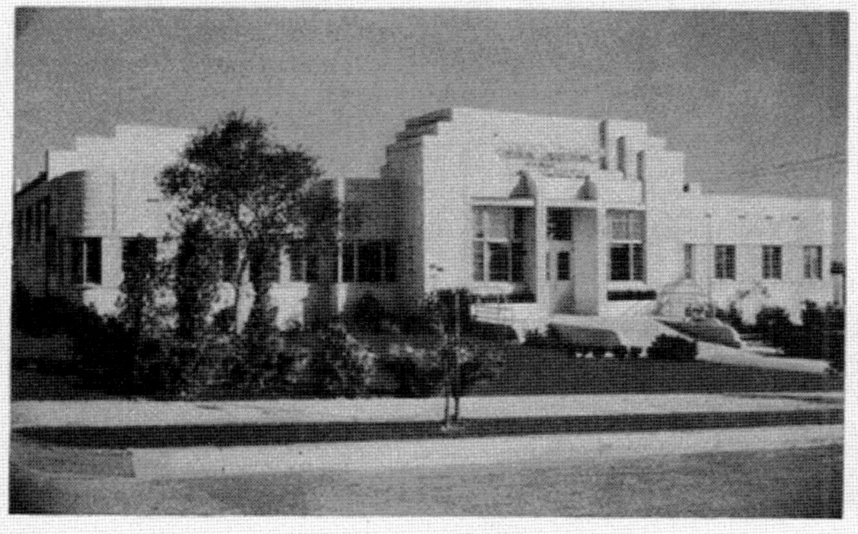

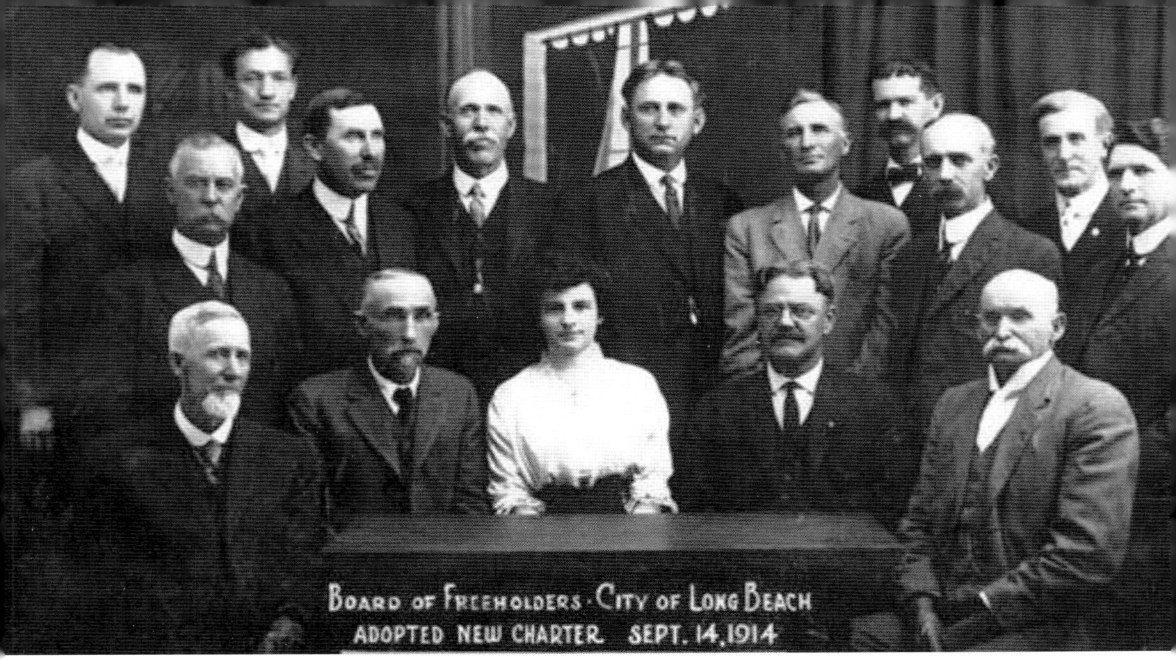
BOARD OF FREEHOLDERS · CITY OF LONG BEACH
ADOPTED NEW CHARTER SEPT. 14, 1914

Above: Local activist and former city staffer, Cora P. Morgan (pictured), appeared before City Council in 1926 concerning problems in the fire department that resulted in the suicide of its fire battalion chief, Jay B. Taylor. She also confronted Mayor Fillmore Condit and accused that the physicians on the hospital board were being personally enriched. Morgan claimed that "instead of being a public institution, fostered by the city, numerous physicians were stockholders of the hospital." Condit stood up and shouted back "you are a liar." After fifty men rose to their feet and yelled "throw him out the window," Condit apologized to Morgan. (*LBPL*)

Below: In anticipation of the traffic that would come to the newly built Marine Stadium during the 1932 Olympics, the city constructed the Alamitos Traffic Circle in 1930. The roundabout was located just below the hill where Community Hospital sat. The circle has been the site of countless automobile accidents whose victims became patients at the hospital. (*CHLBF*)

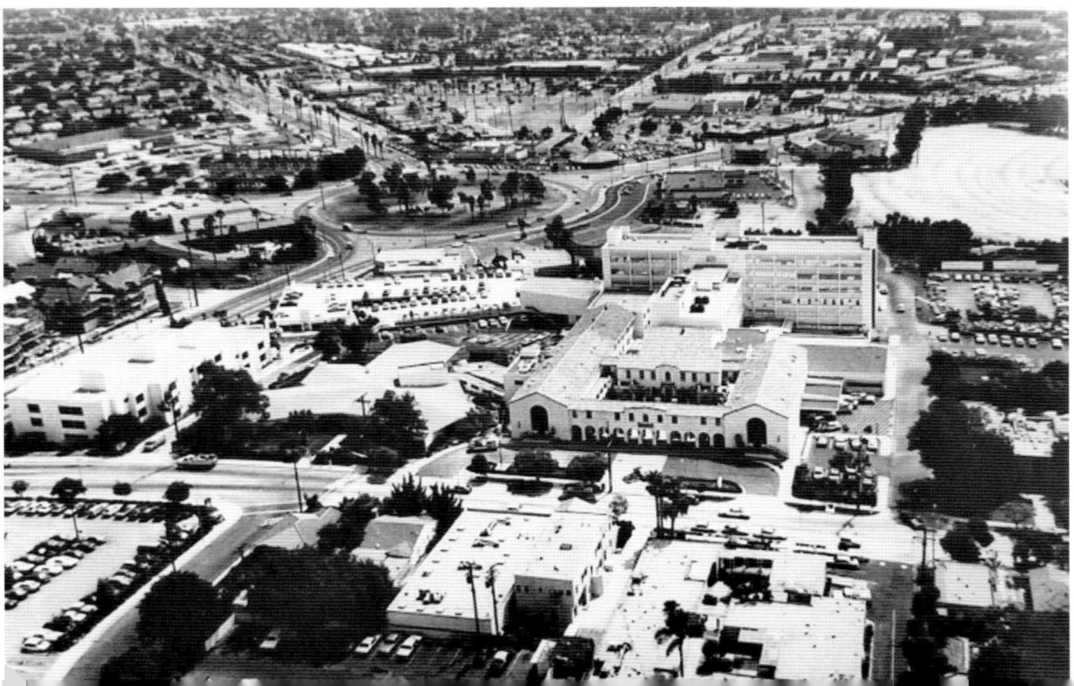

HERE'S CHANCE FOR FREE BABY

Long Beach Institution Will Care Gratis for Infants Born Hospital Day

LONG BEACH, May 8.—In observing Hospital Day, Thursday the 12th inst., the Long Beach Community Hospital, upon recommendation of a staff member, will give free maternity service for five days to mothers whose babies are born on Hospital Day, it was announced today.

Open house will be held Thursday. The Woman's Music Club will give a program which includes a solo by Mrs. Edward W. Green and a piano number by Mrs. Georgia W. Buckingham. The Junior Girls' Glee Club of Woodrow Wilson High School, directed by Edith Hitchcock, will be heard.

In 1932, Community advertised that mothers delivering on Hospital Day could have a "chance for free baby." Upon recommendation of a staff member, the mother could be given five free days of maternity care. (*CHLB*)

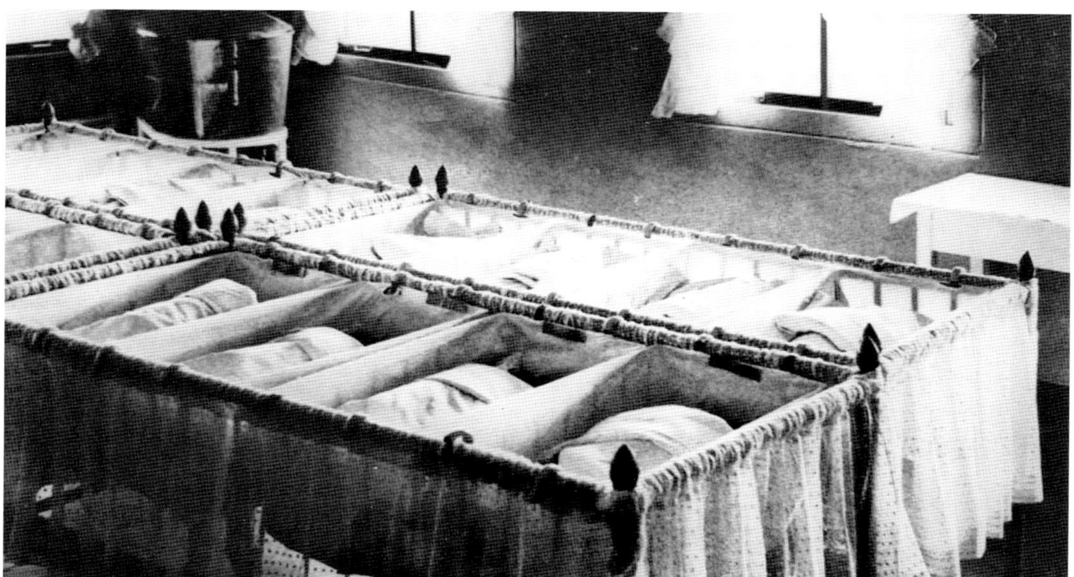

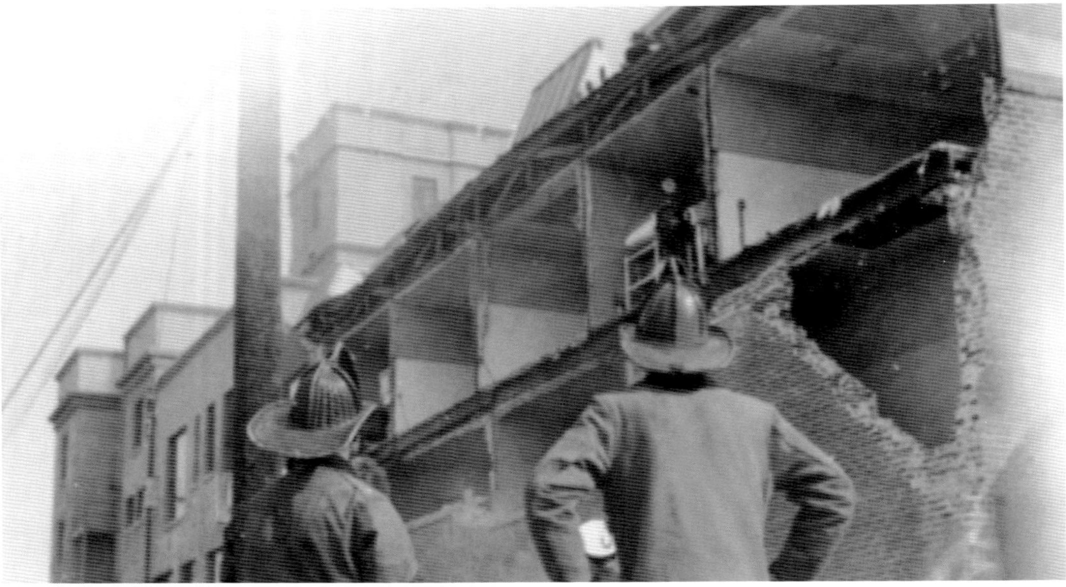

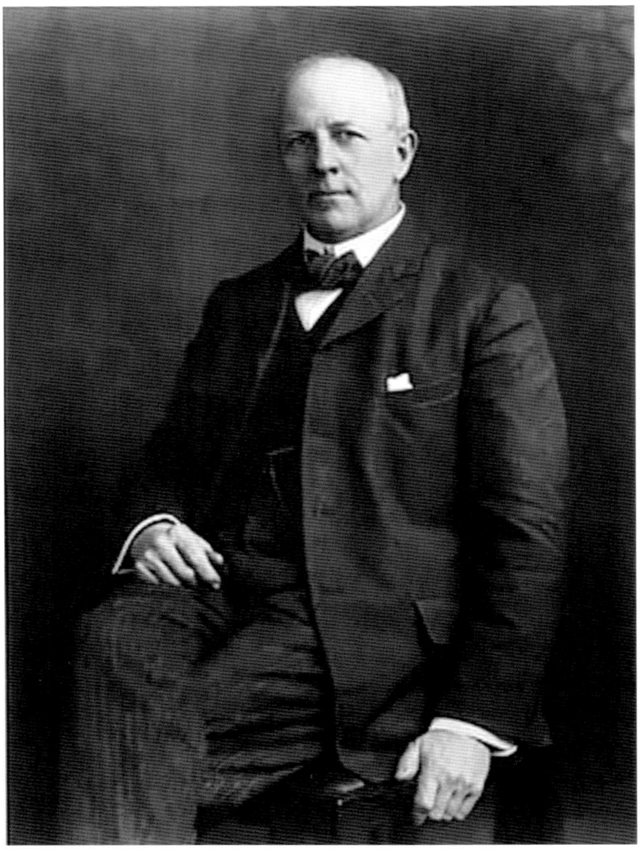

Above: On March 10, 1933, a 6.4 earthquake struck the Newport-Inglewood fault causing considerable damage to buildings. One hundred twenty people died (fifty-two in Long Beach), including five students in the Wilson High School gym, a motorcycle police officer, a firefighter, and a librarian. Community Hospital withstood the shaking and consequently took in most of the injured. More than ninety percent of Long Beach schools were devastated and could not be re-occupied for two years. (*CHLBF*)

Left: "The Father of Community Hospital" passed away at the hospital in 1939 at age eighty-three. Condit never went to formal school but spent his life reading and self-educating up until the end. One newspaper account reported that Condit had just ordered several books so that he could learn Spanish. (*CHLBF*)

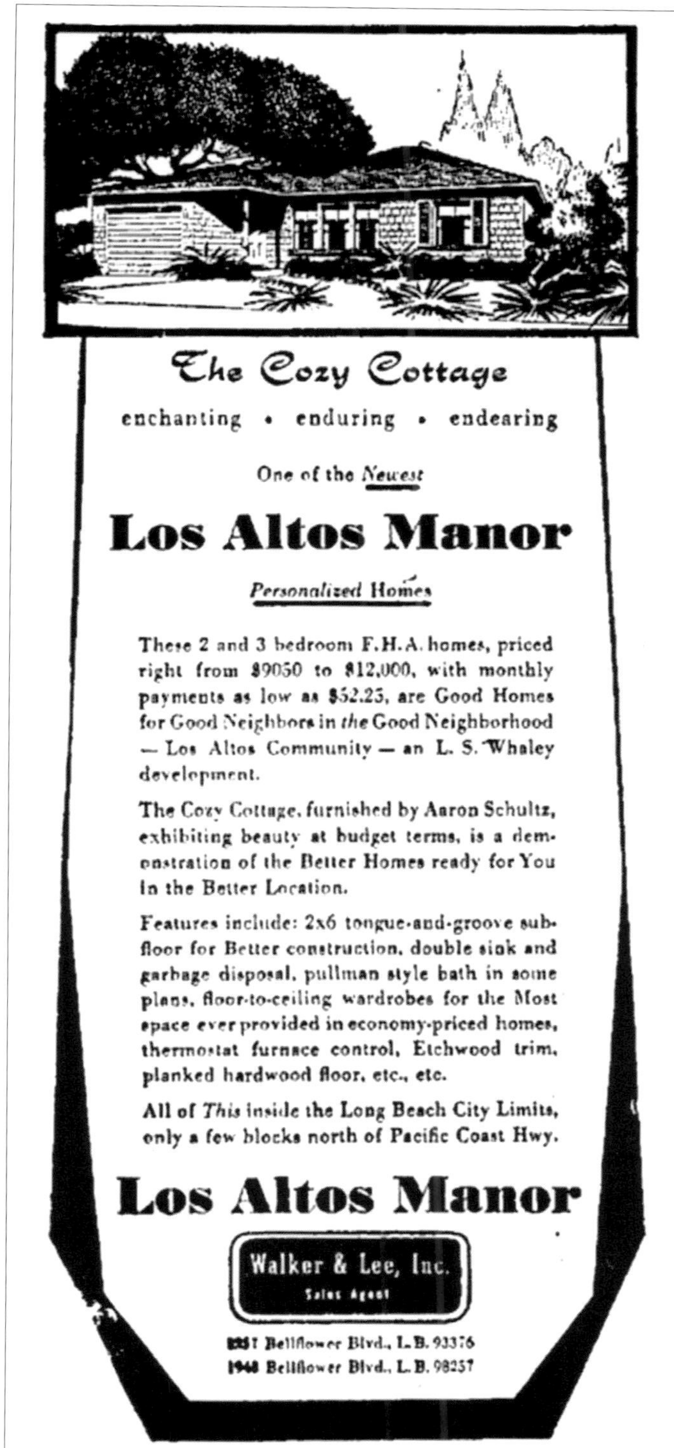

When WWII ended, thousands of new homes were constructed in the Lakewood-Los Altos area because of the number of veterans who could purchase homes without a down payment. This growth brought more babies and a need for an expanded hospital. The photograph shows early Los Altos at the intersections of Bellflower Boulevard and Stearns Avenue. (*LAPL*)

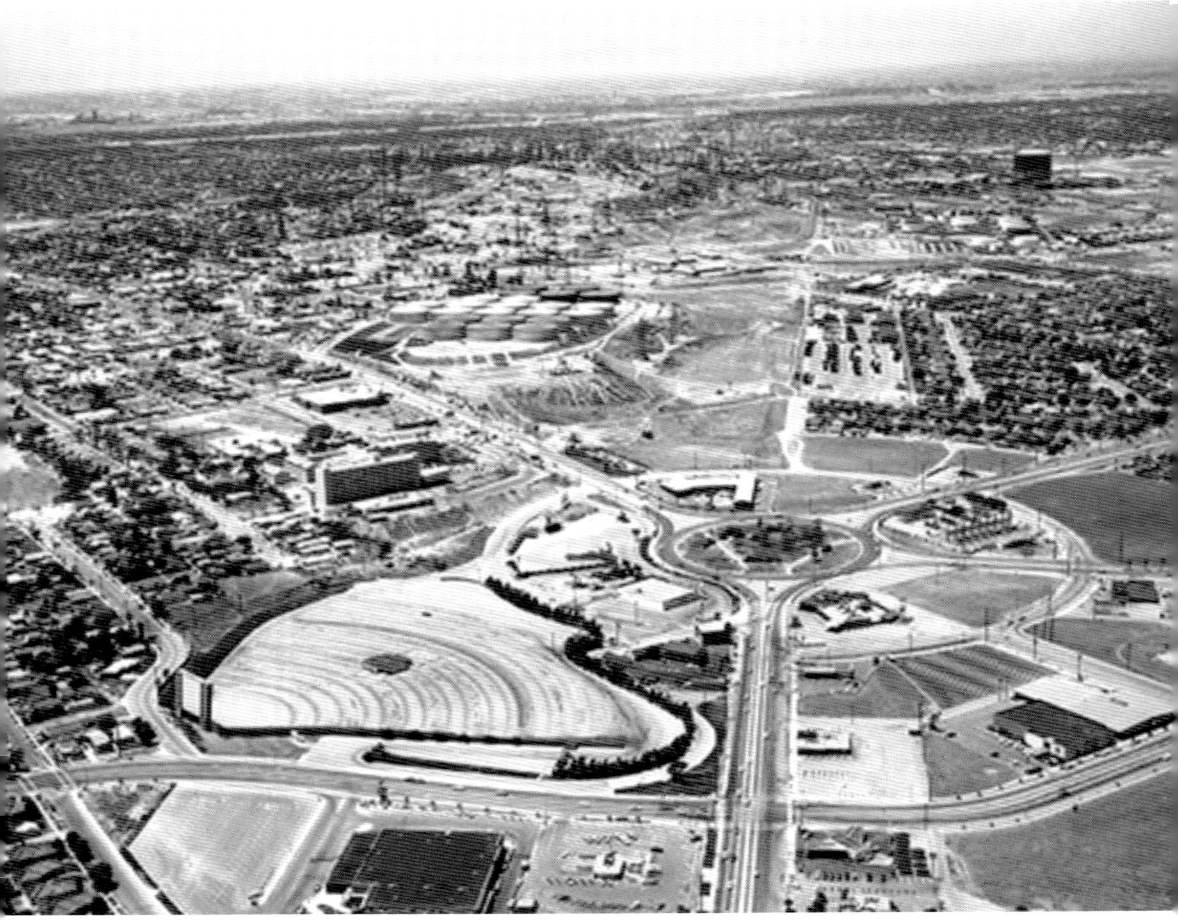

When the new "convalescent unit" and the 1959 expansion were constructed, the hospital patients had a perfect view out of the wide-glass windows to watch movies at the outdoor Circle Drive-In theater (lower left). Community installed speakers in 1960 so that patients could also hear the latest movies. (*CHLBF*)

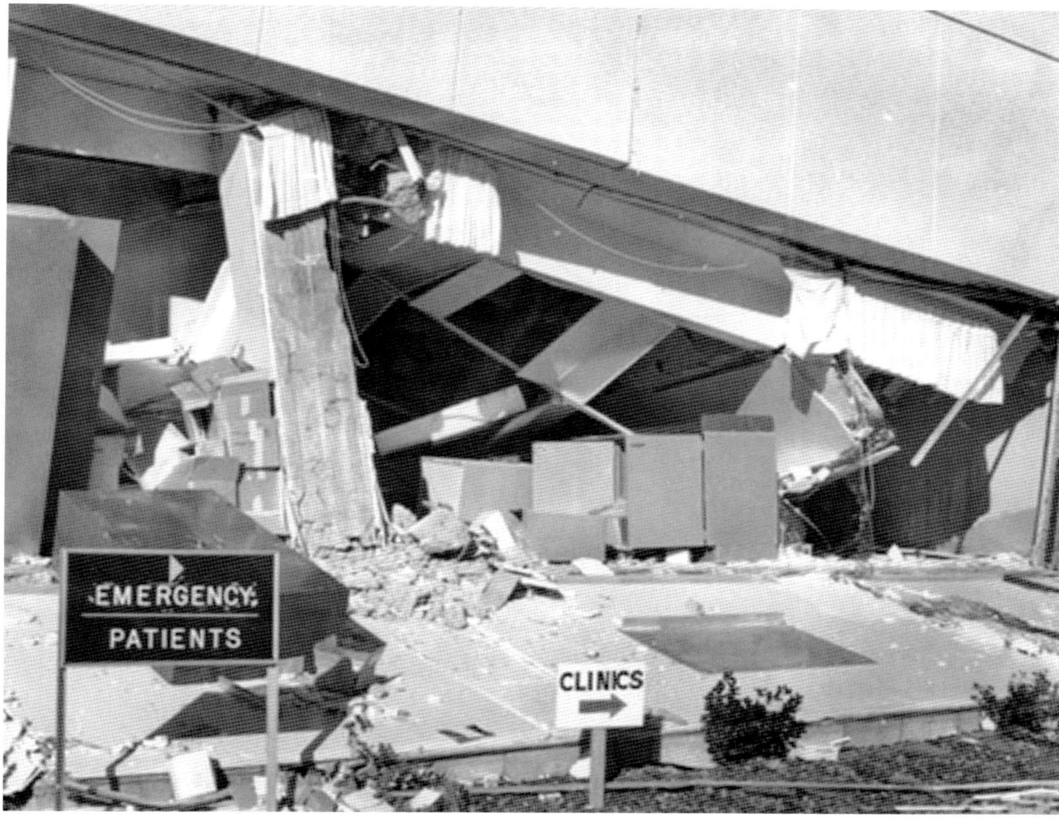

Above: The earthquakes of 1971 (shown in picture) and 1994 resulted in major damage to several Southern California hospitals. The State Legislature then passed requirements that hospitals assess their facilities. In 2001, it was reported that approximately forty percent of California's hospitals buildings "are at risk of collapse in a major earthquake." Hospitals were required to report to the state what they planned to do about their buildings. (*USGS*)

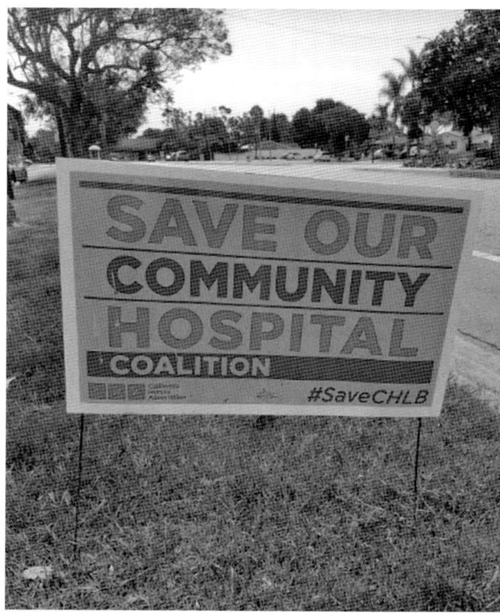

Right: State reports show that nine sections of the hospital are considered "HAZUS fail" due to being located on a fault. The future of this historic hospital is unknown as the "Save Our Community Hospital Coalition" fights to keep the facility open.

7

Osteopathic Hospitals

> Some day when it is more fully understood, osteopathy, as a scientific truth and as a system of treating disease, is going to be prized as a most typical American institution.
>
> *Osteopathy: What it offers as a system of health and profession*, 1920

Osteopathy has a long tradition in Long Beach. Amy (Cook) Rowse, the first woman to marry in Long Beach in 1894, became an osteopath in 1903 after her husband's untimely death.

Although the State of California licensed osteopaths since 1922, the medical profession would not accept them as equals and fought against their practice in hospitals. The Long Beach Community Hospital Association would not allow osteopaths to practice in the new hospital and the City Council would not let an osteopath serve as public health officer. However, the residents of early Long Beach still utilized osteopaths so much so that in 1932, the first osteopathic hospital in Long Beach opened. The Pacific Clinic Hospital provided care for 127 patients, including twenty-eight births in its first year.

The Magnolia Osteopathic Hospital opened in 1934 with eighteen beds. More beds were added in 1940 and 1941. The hospital treated over 1,200 patients a year with more than 200 births. The hospital, operated by osteopathic doctor, Charles Poitevin, closed in 1952.

In 1937, the Bixby Knolls Osteopathic Maternity Hospital was built at 3833 Atlantic Avenue. It was renamed in 1951 as Bixby Knolls Community Hospital. The hospital provided surgical and medical care until 1962 when it was closed after its owner, Dr. Jerome Rehman, was indicted and convicted of charges that he had performed unnecessary operations and failed to observe "sanitary procedures" at the hospital. The building currently is used as space for offices.

As osteopaths grew in numbers and popularity, they added facilities in Long Beach. In 1944, the Long Beach Osteopathic Hospital Association voted to operate Los Cerritos Maternity Hospital at 4005 American Avenue (Virginia Road). By 1945, they were delivering 3,500 babies a year. Los Cerritos was the first to provide post-maternity care in patients' homes. The Osteopathic Association also opened the Long Beach Polyclinic in 1947 to care for people unable to pay private doctors.

The City of Long Beach continued to take in millions of dollars in tidelands oil revenues. All three hospitals—Seaside, St. Mary's and Community—asked for funding to expand their hospitals. In 1952, voters approved a resolution authorizing use of tidelands oil funds for hospitals. The use of tidelands funds was challenged in the California Supreme Court. Voters approved a 10-million-dollar bond issue for hospitals in 1956.

The Long Beach Osteopathic Hospital Association also petitioned the City Council, not for expansion, but for construction of an osteopathic hospital to be located at Pacific and Pine and 27th and 28th. The Association asked for 1.8 million dollars to build a ninety-two-bed hospital designed by Hugh M. Davies. The hospital later renamed "Pacific," opened on June 12, 1956. In 1959, bond revenues were distributed to the hospitals and the Osteopathic Hospital received $1,280,000.

In 1957, medical doctors and osteopaths demonstrated they could work together by launching a joint effort in Long Beach to provide "inoculations" against polio at clinics in St. Mary's, Seaside, Community and the Osteopathic (Pacific) hospitals. Shots were given for free to people who could not pay the three dollars charged by local doctors.

Ironically, just four years later, California voters approved Proposition 22, which stopped the issuance of licenses to "Doctors of Osteopathy." Osteopaths were given the option of becoming an M.D. by paying $65 to the Board of Medical Examiners. The issue was taken to the California Supreme Court. On March 19, 1974, the California Supreme Court ruled unanimously that Proposition 22 was unconstitutional and that D.O.s could be licensed separately from M.D.s. Today, a D.O. receives the same training as an M.D., with added courses in osteopathy.

Pacific Hospital was expanded in 1961 with a ten-bed ICU unit and a 150-seat auditorium. Two convalescent hospitals across the street from the hospital were purchased in 1970. At the same time Pacific was expanding, it was experiencing lower bed occupancy and reduced reimbursements from insurance companies.

In 1997, Pacific was purchased by Health Smart Pacific, Inc. Shortly thereafter, the hospital became embroiled in a fraud scheme in which Pacific Hospital billed insurers more than $580 million for spinal surgeries on over 4,400 patients. Insurers paid the hospital more than $226 million for the surgeries performed because of illegal kickbacks. The hospital was closed and then reopened in 2013 as "College Medical Center."

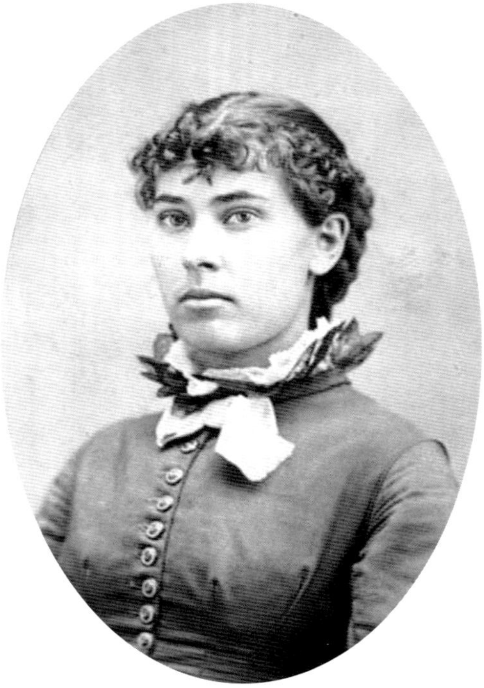

Amy (Cook) Rowse was the first woman to be married in the new city of Long Beach in 1894. She became an osteopath in 1903 after the untimely death of her husband. (*LBPL*)

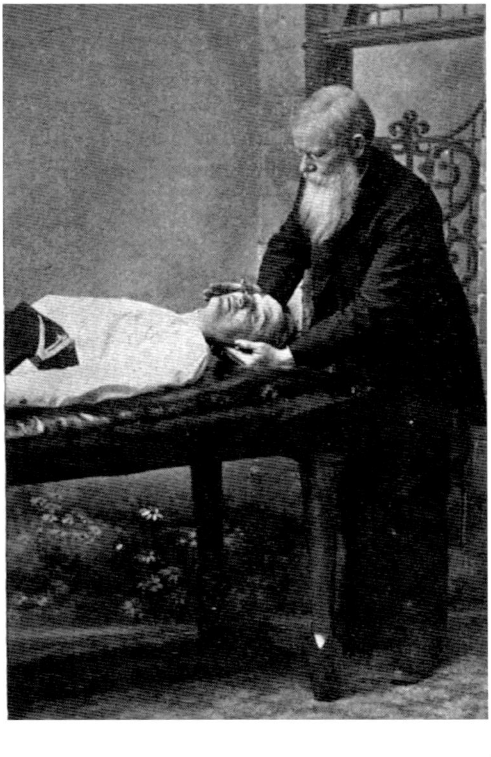

Left: The first osteopathic hospital in Long Beach opened in 1932 at 1036 Pacific Avenue. Early osteopaths utilized treatments that did not rely upon medicine, but manipulations as shown here in the 1899 *Osteopathy Illustrated*. Osteopaths considered themselves to be "pioneers" in drugless healthcare and sometimes referred to their degree, D.O., as "dig on."

Opposite: Adjacent to Long Beach in the then-unincorporated area called "Signal Hill" stood "Dr. Pikes Osteopathic Health Resort" as shown in the 1920 edition of *The Western Osteopath*.

DR. PIKE'S
Osteopathic Health Resort

2639 Wall Street, bet. Temple and Dakota Aves.

SIGNAL HILL, LONG BEACH

R. F. D. 3, Box 820

DIRECTIONS—Autos take East Anaheim Blvd. to Temple Ave. north to Wall St. Or take Willowville via Zaferia car, and get off at Temple Station. From Los Angeles take Newport car, get off at Temple Station.

ACCOMMODATIONS—Ample grounds of 8 acres, elevation nearly 200 feet. Modern two-room cottages, and all-weather **Canvas-Houses.** Milk diet and rest cure. Scientific health meals with our usual combination treatments, i. e., Sun, Radium, Mineral Baths, Electric Blanket.

KIND OF CASES TREATED Mental, Nervous and Constitutional Diseases, also Digestive Disorders.

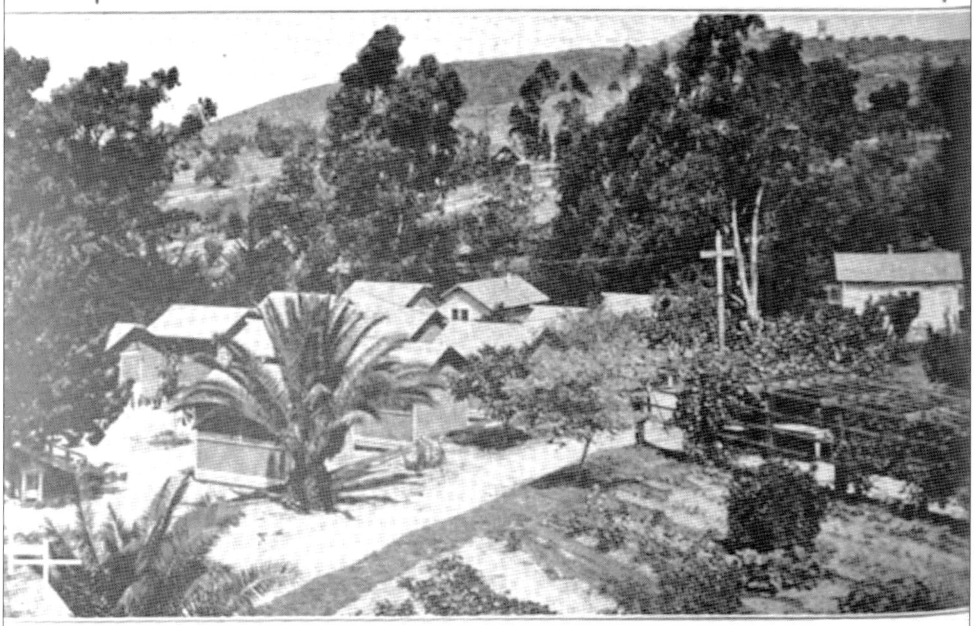

Dr. Pike's Osteopathic Health Resort

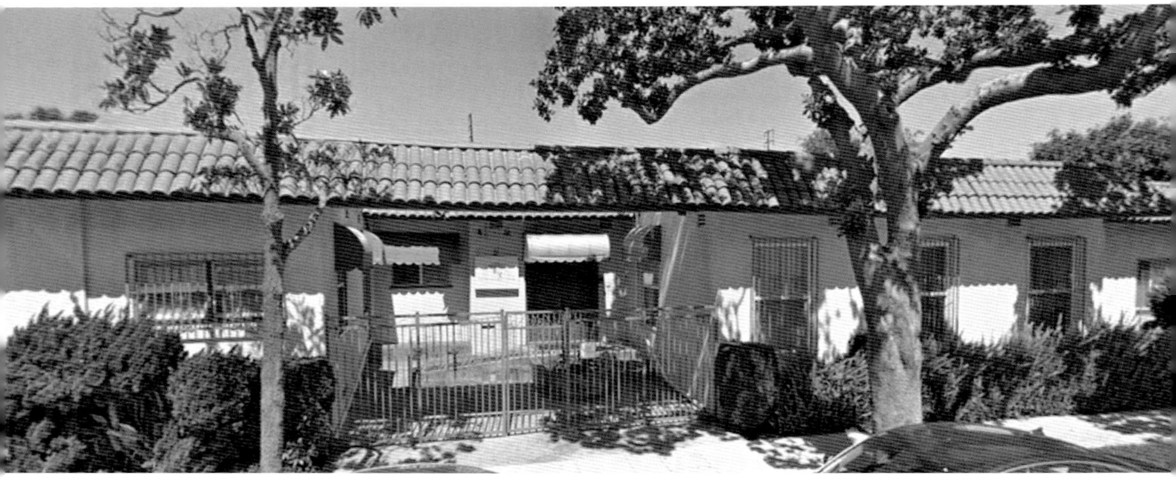

The Magnolia Osteopathic Hospital opened at 2101 Magnolia Avenue in 1934 with eighteen beds and expanded in 1940 and 1961. Today, the building houses the Tarzana Treatment Center for drug and alcohol addiction.

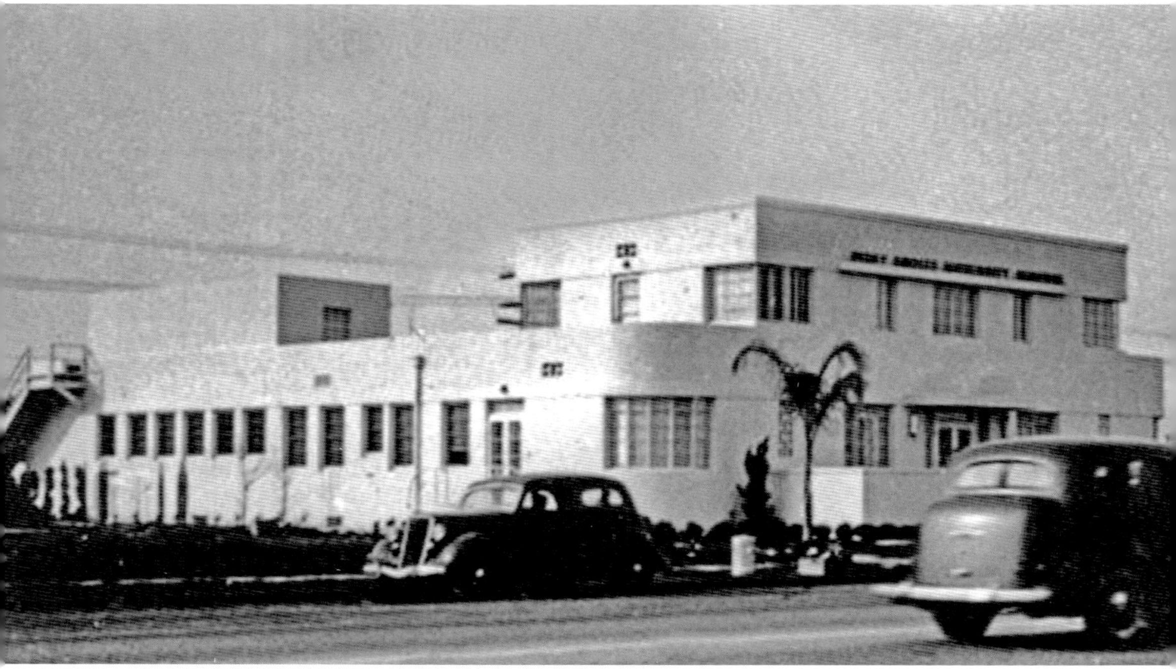

The Bixby Knolls Osteopathic Maternity Hospital opened in 1937 at 3833 Atlantic Avenue, as one of several facilities providing maternity care in the city. It was renamed in 1951 as Bixby Knolls Community Hospital. (*LBPL*)

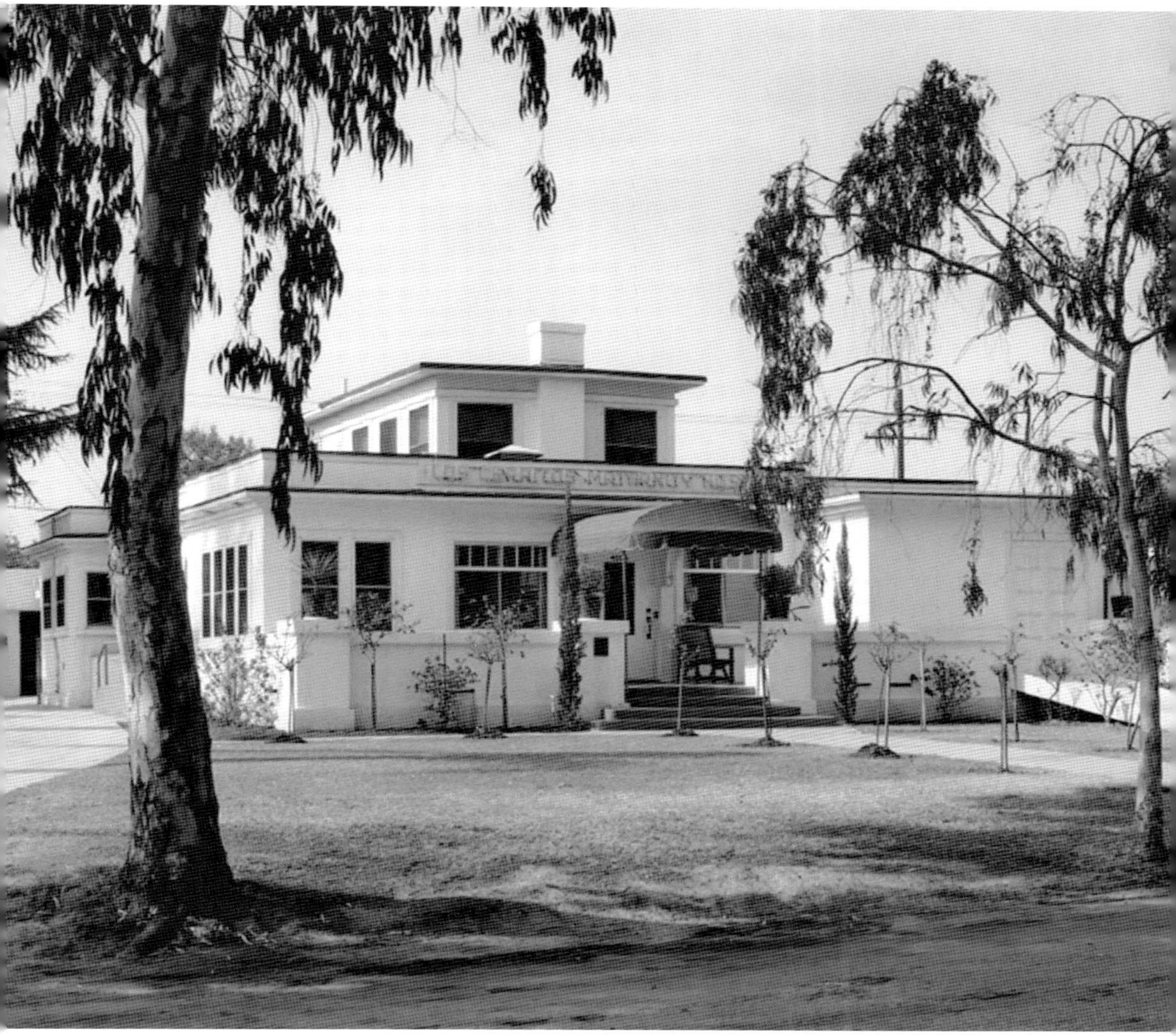

Pictured is the Los Cerritos Maternity Hospital at 4005 American Avenue (Virginia Road). By 1945, they were delivering 3,500 babies a year. (*HSLB*)

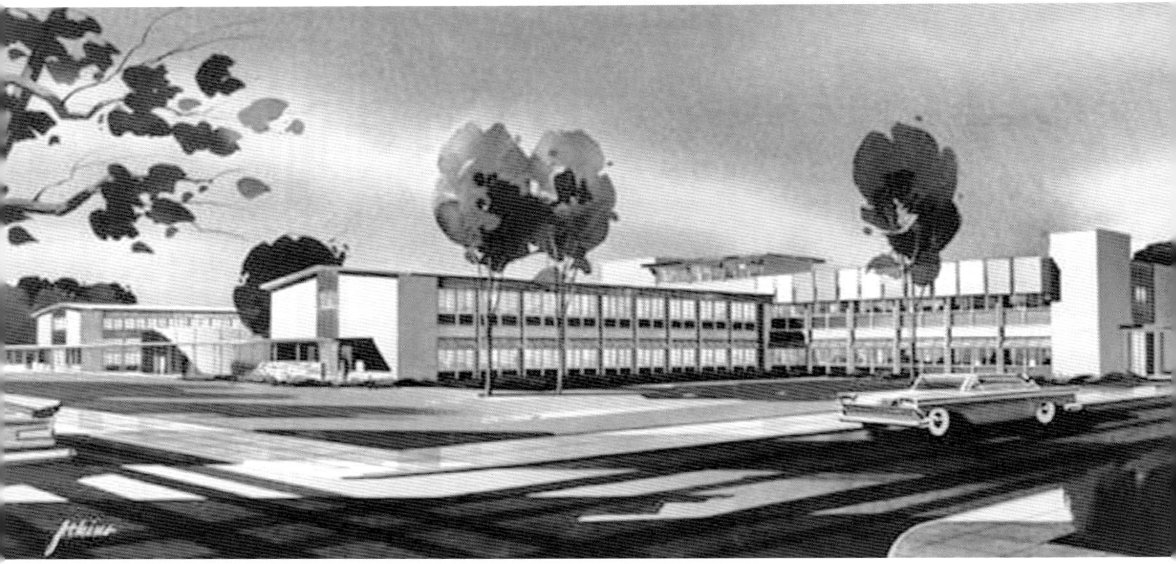

The Long Beach Osteopathic Hospital Association petitioned the City Council for 1.8 million dollars in tidelands oil funds for the construction of a ninety-two-bed osteopathic hospital. The photograph shows the architectural drawings. (*LBPL*)

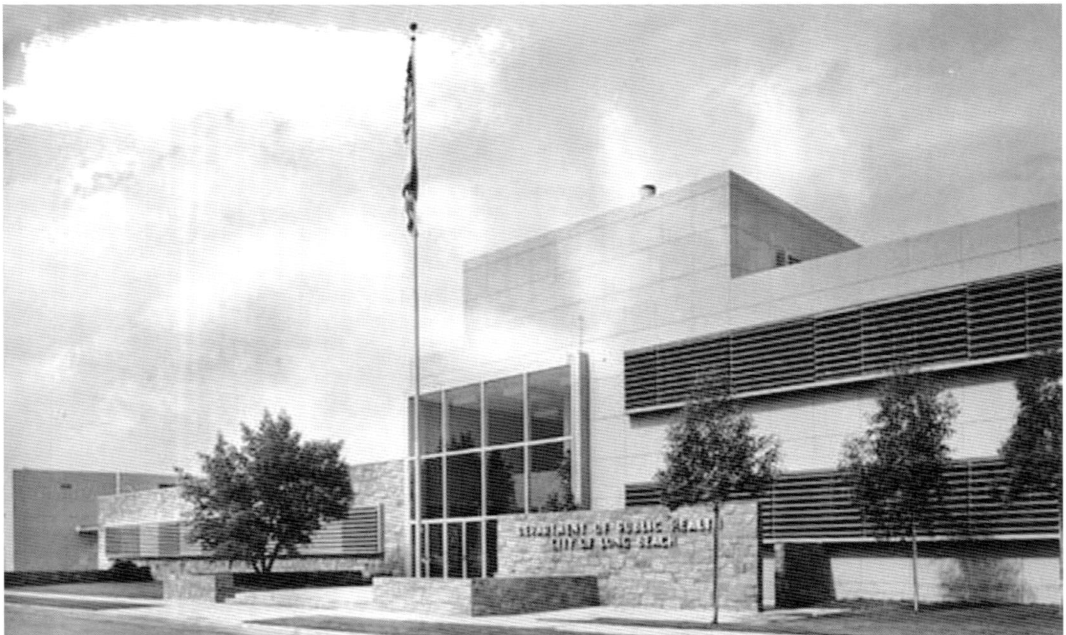

The City of Long Beach located its health department adjacent to Pacific Hospital. The city health department was re-located in the 1990s, to 2525 Grand Avenue. (*LBPL*)

8

MILITARY, VETERAN AND COUNTY HOSPITALS

To care for him who shall have borne the battle, and for his widow, and his orphan.

Words of U.S. President Abraham Lincoln used as Mission Statement of U.S. Veterans Administration

From the early 1900s, Long Beach officials lobbied the United States Navy to port ships there. In 1908, a portion of "the Great White Fleet" came to Long Beach as part of its world-wide tour to show the strength of the U.S. When the city dedicated its Lincoln statue in 1915, the secretary of the Navy sent a ship to provide a twenty-one-gun salute.

The Navy sent its first two aircraft carriers, the USS *Lexington* and USS *Saratoga*, to anchor off the coast of Long Beach while conducting flying exercises in 1928. The Navy added more ships at Long Beach. Many of the ships destroyed or severely damaged during the December 7, 1941, attack on Pearl Harbor had been ported in Long Beach.

The U.S. Naval Dry Docks and Roosevelt Base were built in 1943, bringing thousands of military personnel and their families to Long Beach. Construction of a Naval hospital began December 6, 1941, on a 100-acre site on the grounds of Alamitos Rancho (7th Street and Bellflower Boulevard). During construction, a "mysterious fire" ravaged part of the hospital. It opened in December 1942. By 1945, the hospital was at full capacity with 3,913 patients. The hospital employed 430 civilian and 750 military personnel.

During the war, a "Ferry Command Station Hospital" was located on 30 acres at Willow Street and Newport Avenue in Signal Hill. In 1948, the hospital was converted into Los Angeles County "Long Beach General Hospital." It included twenty-two buildings. The first patients were admitted to a twenty-five-bed tuberculosis unit. General Hospital expanded and provided services to paralyzed, elderly and alcoholic patients. The county closed the facility in 1984. The facility was demolished, and the land turned into a "business park."

When Seaside Hospital was sold to Los Angeles County, part of it was utilized as El Cerrito hospital. When the Long Beach General Hospital closed, many patients were transferred to outpatient clinics at El Cerrito until the county built the Comprehensive Center Health Center in the late 1980s.

After WWII, the Navy announced that it would close the Long Beach Naval Hospital by June 1950. The city and medical community lobbied intensely to keep the hospital open, arguing that its closure would devastate the economy. Others lobbied that the hospital be given to the Veterans Administration.

City officials had argued since the late 1920s that the good weather and climate were attracting more and more veterans from across the country and that a veterans' facility was needed.

On June 1, 1950, the Navy officially transferred the hospital to the U.S. Veterans Administration. More than 1,200 patients were transferred from the VA hospital in Van Nuys, which was closing. The VA announced it would utilize 1,600 beds and employ 2,200. The Navy anchored the hospital ship USS *Haven* off the coast to provide 350 beds for military personnel. Today, the Long Beach VA is one of the finest medical centers in the VA system.

Long Beach continued to lobby for a new Naval hospital and offered to give the Navy 30.5 acres at the north end of El Dorado Park for $10. Construction started in the spring of 1965 and the hospital was commissioned on February 1, 1967. Captain H. Von Radesky was appointed the first administrative officer.

The five-story Naval hospital designed by local architects, Don and Hugh Gibbs, cost over 7 million dollars. As the causalities of the Vietnam War increased, additional beds were needed. To assist, the hospital ship USS *Repose* was anchored nearby. It was estimated that the hospital would serve 200,000 military dependents and retired military in the greater Long Beach area.

In 1994, the Navy closed both the Naval Shipyard and the Naval Hospital. The city was given the property, which it used to develop the "Towne Center," a multi-store shopping area.

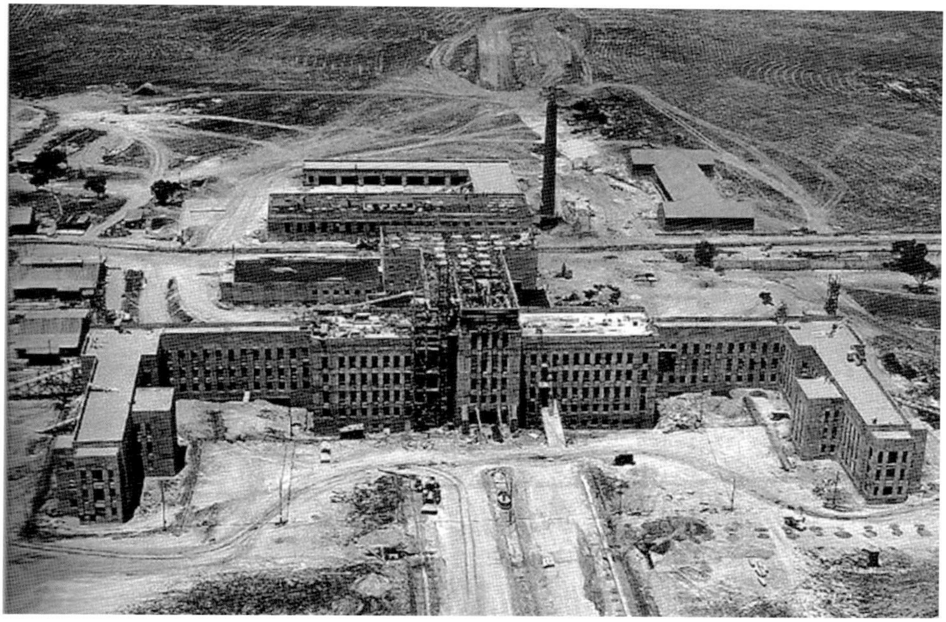

Above and below: Most of the ships destroyed or damaged in Pearl Harbor in 1941 had been ported in Long Beach. The Naval Hospital was completed in 1943 and was located at 7th Street and Bellflower Boulevard, on land once lived on by the Tongva. (*US Naval Medicine*)

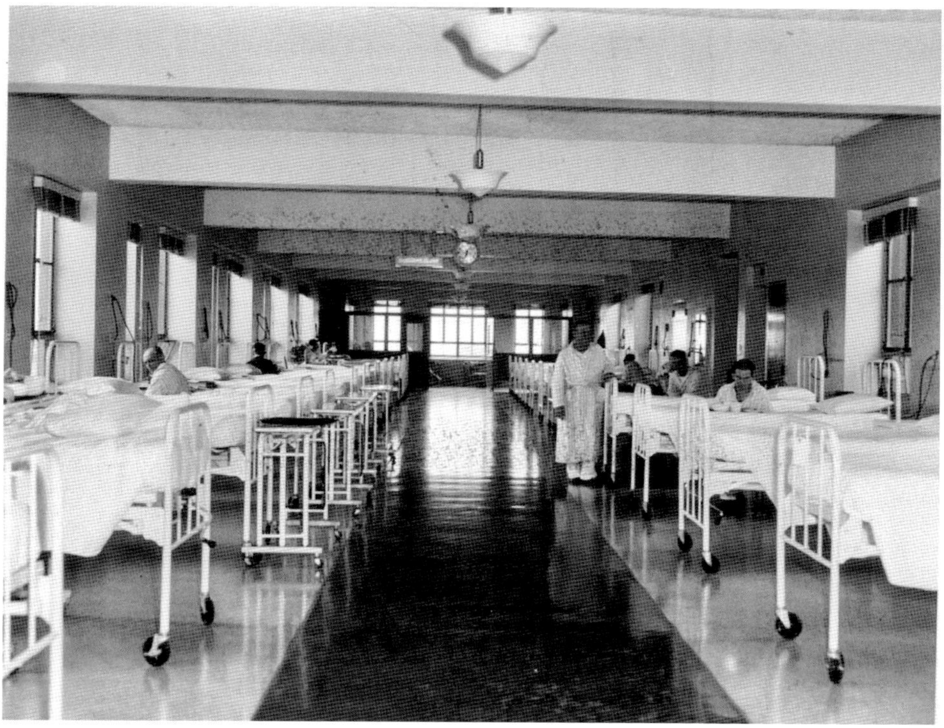

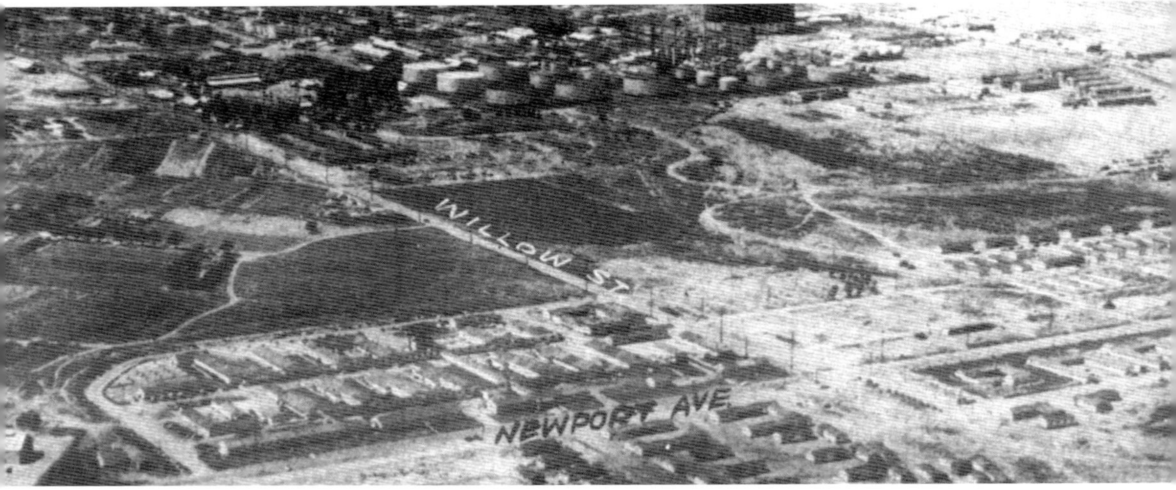

The Long Beach General Hospital site is shown in this 1948 photograph. The site was the former "Ferry Command Station Hospital." The 6th Ferrying Group of the Army's Air Transport Command was stationed nearby at the Long Beach airfield. Planes built by Douglas Aircraft Plant were "ferried" to military bases for use in WWII.

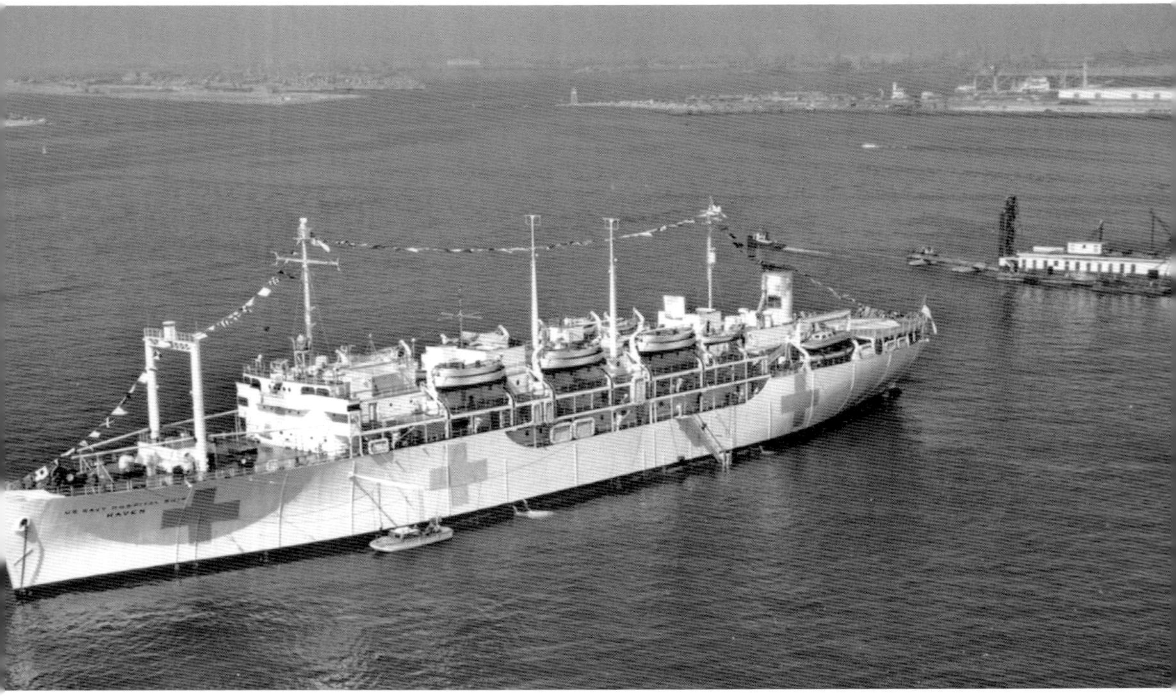

The entire Long Beach Naval hospital property was converted to a VA hospital in 1950. The hospital ship, USS *Haven*, anchored off Long Beach in 1957 to take care of military patients because the area no longer had a military hospital. (*USNA*)

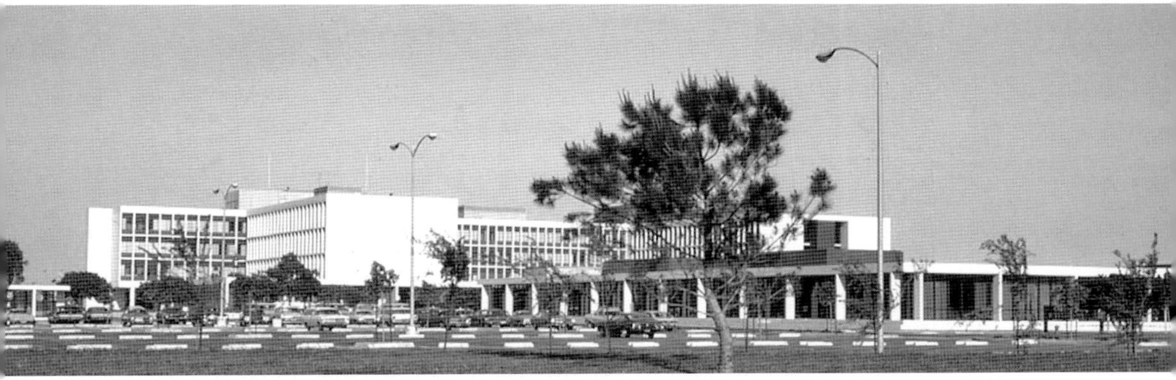

The new LB Naval Hospital was designated Naval Regional Medical Center in 1972. During the Vietnam war, the hospital and hospital ship USS *Repose* served as primary point for personnel returning via air medical evacuation. (*USNA*)

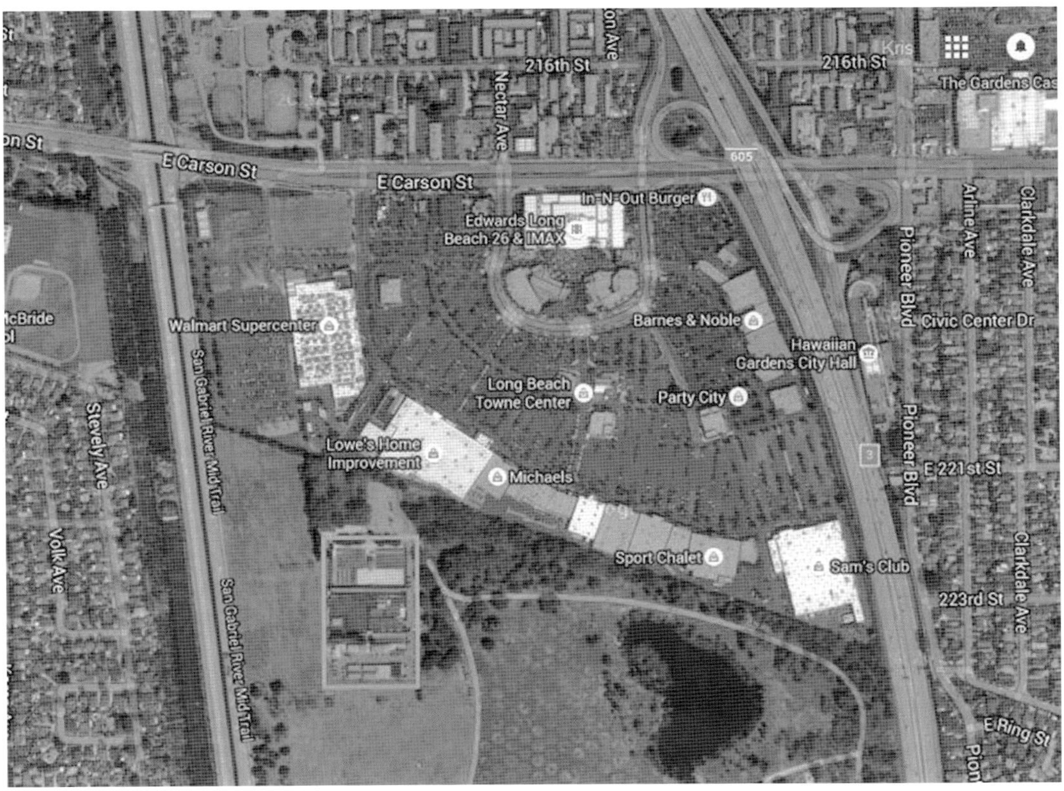

The Navy closed the Naval Shipyard and the Naval Hospital in 1992. One section of the hospital property was sold to Vestar Development and the other, quitclaimed to the City of Long Beach. A major shopping complex called the "Towne Center" was built on both sections. A police academy was also added to the property as outlined in this photograph.

9

Early Long Beach Faces Medical Emergencies

> The purpose of government is to protect its citizens, and a government which fails to shelter its citizens against infection is neither intelligent nor moral.
>
> February 18, 1922, California State Board of Health Weekly Bulletin

Early Long Beach faced many of the same healthcare problems of any growing city and more because it was a seaside resort. The city grappled with communicable diseases, sanitation and sewage, controlling the dust from the roads, automobile and trolley accidents, near drownings at the ocean and sloughs, children's health, access to clean drinking water, abatement of the mosquitoes that filled the wetlands, building collapses and natural disasters.

These healthcare problems were compounded as thousands of visitors came to walk on the pier, swim in the ocean, purchase food from vendors, ride a roller coaster at the Pike or camp on the beach while attending "Encampments" of Civil War veterans or the summer Methodist Chautauqua.

The city government had the foresight to establish a Board of Public Health and a public health officer. It selected a succession of qualified physicians who were keenly aware of the need to actively involve public health in making the city a healthy place in which to live and to visit.

Dr. Harriman Jones served as the city's public health officer from 1904-1910. He is often referred to as the city's "first public health officer," but in fact was the third to serve. Jones perhaps is given that designation because of his many significant and advanced public health initiatives.

He fought to expand the city's sewer system and started the Long Beach Pure Food Commission. A strong advocate for children's health care, Jones insisted there be a "municipal nurse" to care for school children.

Jones made headlines in 1908 when he ordered the Long Beach School Board to require child vaccinations. Jones understood that many communicable diseases could be avoided with proper vaccination. His battle with the local school board went statewide. He and Dr. W. L. Woodruff battled publicly over the issue until it was decided at the state level and all children were required to be vaccinated.

In 1909, a group of Long Beach women founded the Bethlehem Inn at 27 Maine Avenue to provide maternity care for girls. They required the girls to be married to obtain care. Dr. Jones withdrew his financial support when he learned of the requirement and the inn closed.

Jones helped form the Long Beach Hospital during the time he served as public health officer. He then served as a surgeon at the Long Beach Sanitarium. Jones later helped establish Seaside Hospital. In 1930, he purchased land in Signal Hill to build a clinic and hospital. Oil made the land very valuable and he opened Harriman Jones Clinic and Hospital on property owned by Park Nursery on Broadway and Junipero.

Communicable diseases such as tuberculosis, infantile paralysis, smallpox and influenza took their toll in Los Angeles County. Because Long Beach had its own public health staff, it was able to control the outbreak more than the county could.

Today, the Long Beach Health Department annually provides over 350,000 public health visits, 16,000 immunizations, 300,000 food nutrition vouchers, 7,800 food facility inspections, 5,400 miles of spraying for mosquitoes, 2,700 public health nurse visits and 780 recreational water tests. Over 7,000 homeless individuals are assisted with housing and other services.

On November 9, 1906, Long Beach faced its first large-scale medical emergency. The Hotel Bixby, described as "one of the largest reinforced concrete buildings in the world," partly collapsed, injuring several workers and sending ten others to their death as the five floors broke apart. One of the injured, James Walsh, lingered for two months in the Long Beach Hospital before he died from complications of crush injuries. Construction resumed, and the hotel was renamed Hotel Virginia in 1908.

In 1912, infantile paralysis hit Los Angeles County, impacting children more than adults. The Los Angeles County Public Health Department issued orders that children under twelve were not allowed to attend Sunday school and children under fifteen could not attend public meetings or moving picture houses. These orders were issued to stop the spread of the disease. Long Beach City Council went even further in passing an ordinance that prohibited children from amusement parks, picnics and schools. Local businesses complained loudly that since there were no cases of the disease in the city, the council should remove the restrictions. It did in August 1912.

From time to time, the Long Beach public health officer took matters into his own hands to control disease. In 1913, it was reported that the health officer, T.H. Newman, built "with his own hands" a five-foot fence around a house where there was a case of scarlet fever. Because the house was near a school and the post office, Newman did not want children or adults entering the area.

Another major collapse happened on May 24, 1913, during the celebration of Empire Day (Queen Victoria's birthday). More than 20,000 gathered to celebrate. The women, children and elderly men assembled on the municipal pier adjacent to the auditorium. They waited as the men completed their parade down Pine Avenue. Fifty women and children were killed and 200 injured when forty feet of the pier collapsed. Low tide prevented many from drowning as they were thrown to the sand. A makeshift hospital and morgue were set up and bodies placed on the sand. Some of the injured were taken to the Long Beach Sanitarium and Seaside Hospital. The City of Long Beach was sued when it was discovered that the collapse was due to failure to replace rotted support pilings.

The Spanish Flu pandemic of 1918 killed 20 million worldwide. In Long Beach, 3,160 people died of the flu—many of them young children. It was reported that number of deaths would have been higher if the city public health officer had not closed places where people gathered, such as theaters, amusement places, dance halls and movie houses.

No one was immune from the disease. Dr. William J. Cook, who practiced medicine in Long Beach for over thirteen years, was the first physician in the city to die from influenza. Vaccinations were controversial, and the government took every effort to encourage citizens to get a shot against the flu.

In 1919, the city public health officer, Dr. Ralph Taylor, launched an effort to rid the city of mosquitoes. This required draining many acres of lowlands and "spreading of oil over stagnant pools."

Southern California was hit with another type of epidemic in 1929 when thousands of cattle and other animals were infected with "hoof and mouth disease" caused by the Q-fever. Motorcycle police ("quarantine guards") were stationed at the borders of Los Angeles County to keep people from leaving with pets who might have been infected. A Long Beach oil worker was shot by a quarantine guard one evening because of his failure to halt in a restricted area. The Bixby Ranch was ordered to herd thousands of their cattle into mass graves and then shoot them. Japanese hog farmers in Signal Hill had to destroy their pigs. The outbreak was traced back to "contaminated meat scraps" found in the trash hold of a ship docked at the port of Los Angeles. The scraps had been fed to hogs on a farm in Montebello.

On March 10, 1933, at 5:54 p.m., a 6.4-magnitude earthquake struck Long Beach and surrounding communities. An estimated 120 died and countless others were injured, from debris falling from buildings and homes. The earthquake destroyed most of Long Beach schools and damaged both Seaside and St. Mary's hospitals. Community Hospital sustained little damage.

Polio outbreaks increased in frequency during the late 1940s and early 1950s. According to the Centers for Disease Control, polio crippled an average of more than 35,000 people each year. Long Beach public health officials ordered quarantines and prohibited children under sixteen in certain places. All local hospitals held "polio clinics" where residents could get immunizations. Parents kept their children away from the Colorado Lagoon which had been given the title "polio pit."

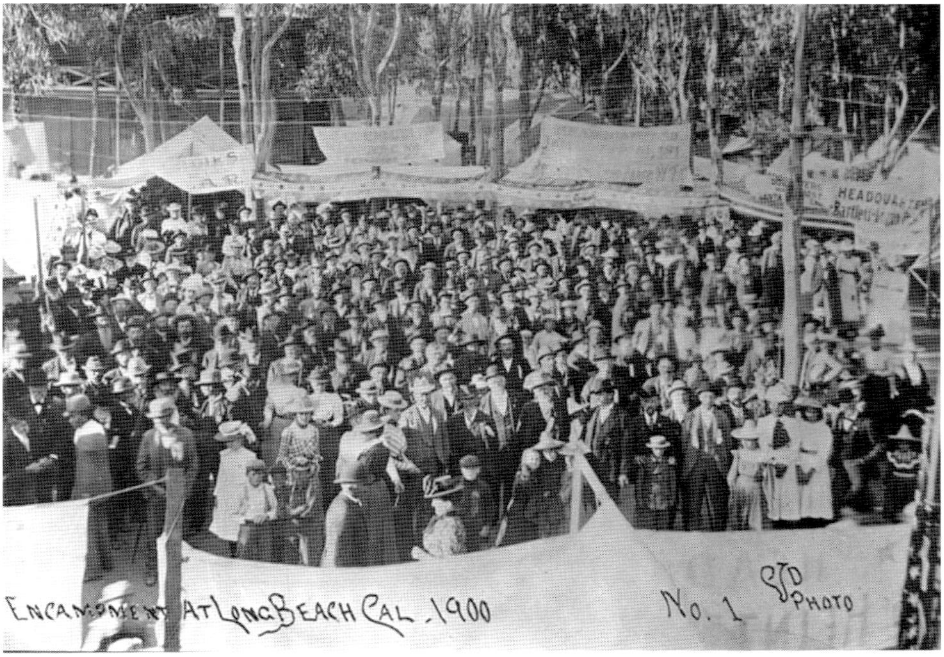

As Civil War veterans moved to Long Beach, the city quickly became the site of annual "Grand Army of the Republic" encampments. These annual meetings drew thousands of visitors, who camped on the beach or in park areas.

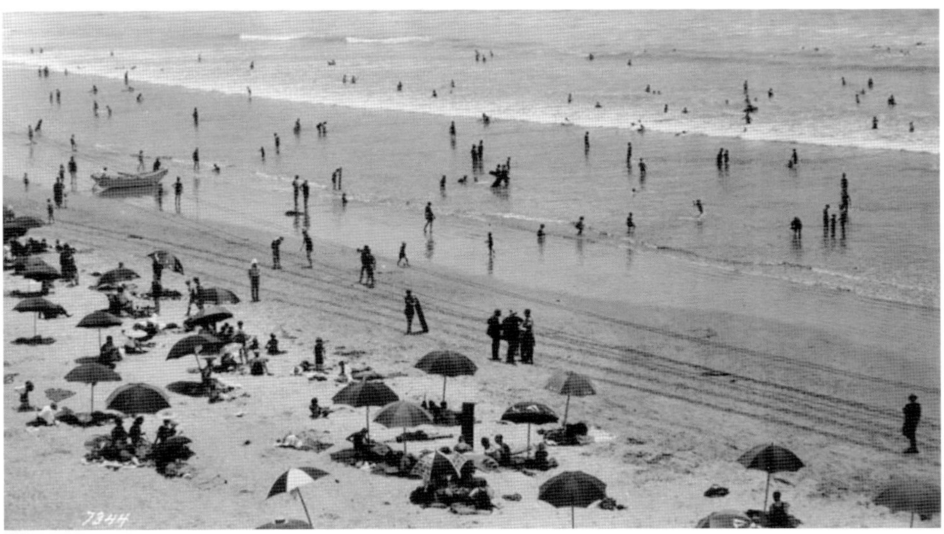

Visitors flocked to the beach and waves in Long Beach. In the early 1900s, so many people died from drowning that national newspapers raised the question of whether the city was criminally negligent for not doing something to save tourists. The city responded by providing lifeguards clad in red suits with boats along the beach (visible in the photograph).

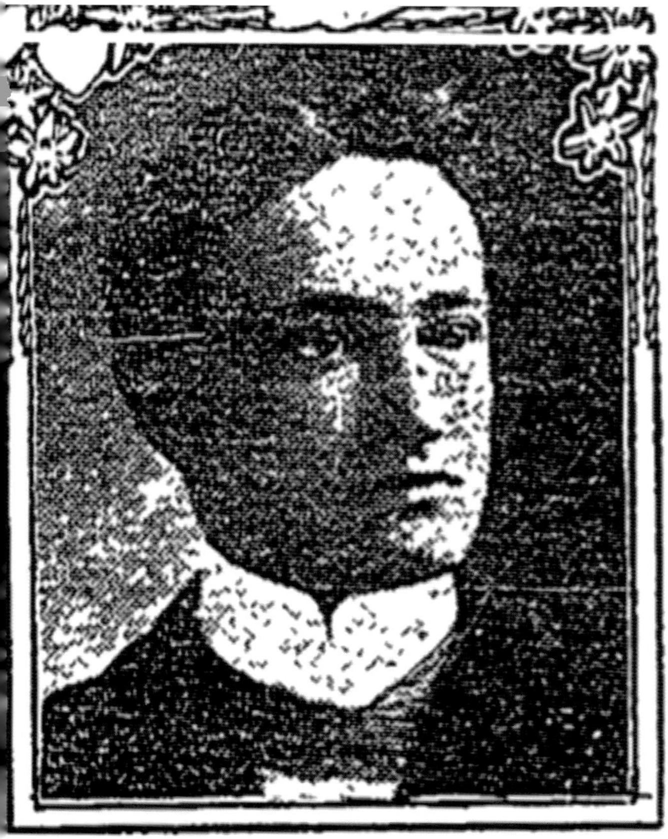

Left: Dr. W. Harriman Jones, a native of Battle Creek, Michigan, came to Long Beach in 1903. Jones was appointed Long Beach public health officer in 1904 and served until 1910. He was responsible for establishing the Long Beach Hospital and served there as a surgeon. He was also a founding member of Seaside Hospital and served for many years as its chief of staff.

Below: Dr. Jones introduced numerous public health regulations and initiatives such as stopping restaurants from dumping garbage on the beach and extending sewers to the northern part of the city. Beginning in 1905, public health officers were required to sign all burial permits and to record the cause of deaths.

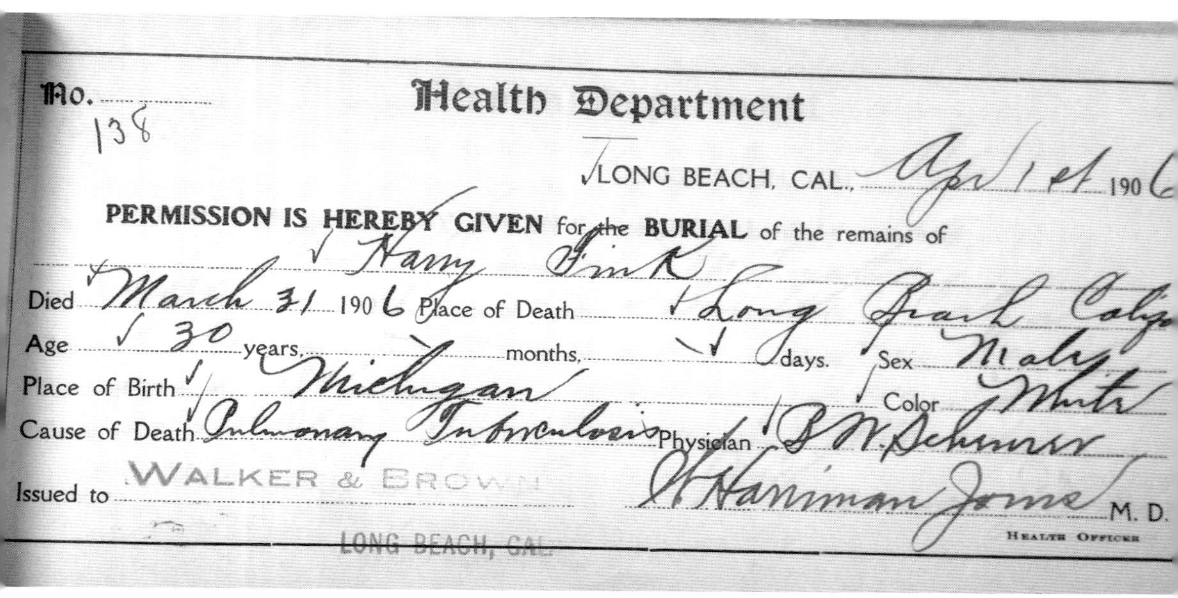

No. 138

Health Department

LONG BEACH, CAL., Apl 1st 1906

PERMISSION IS HEREBY GIVEN for the **BURIAL** of the remains of Harry Fink

Died March 31 1906 Place of Death Long Beach Calif

Age 30 years, months, days. Sex Male

Place of Birth Michigan Color White

Cause of Death Pulmonary Tuberculosis Physician B N Schreiner

Issued to WALKER & BROWN LONG BEACH, CAL.

W Harriman Jones M. D.
HEALTH OFFICER

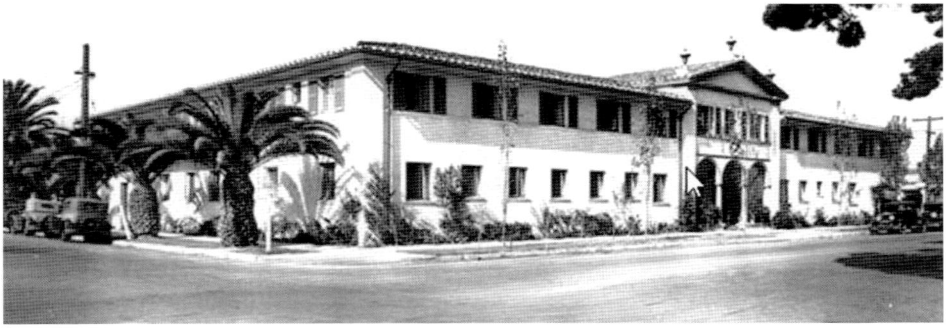

In the 1930s, Dr. Jones established the forty-seven-bed Harriman Jones Clinic and Hospital located at Broadway and Cherry Avenue. Jones put a clinic within a hospital as a way of lowering costs. He practiced medicine until 1956. The hospital portion of the facility closed in 1964. His clinic was designated a "historic landmark" of the City of Long Beach in 1989. Today, a Rite Aid leases the property. (*LBPL*)

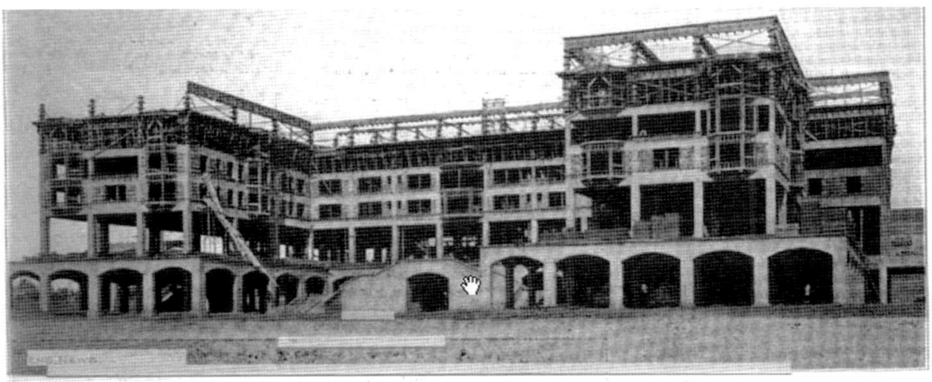

FIG. 1. VIEW OF HOTEL BIXBY, LONG BEACH, CAL., UNDER CONSTRUCTION OF REINFORCED CONCRETE.
(View Taken from Sea Front Oct. 25, 1906.)

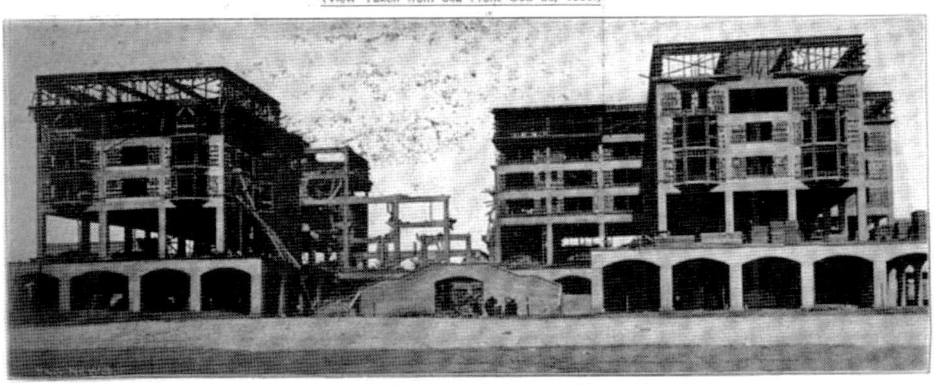

FIG. 2. VIEW OF HOTEL BIXBY AFTER COLLAPSE OF NOV. 9, 1906.

The first serious medical emergency faced by the City of Long Beach was in 1906 when five floors of the Hotel Bixby collapsed during construction. The collapse was the topic of many "engineering journals" who were concerned about reinforced concrete. The hotel was quietly renamed Hotel Virginia and opened in 1908.

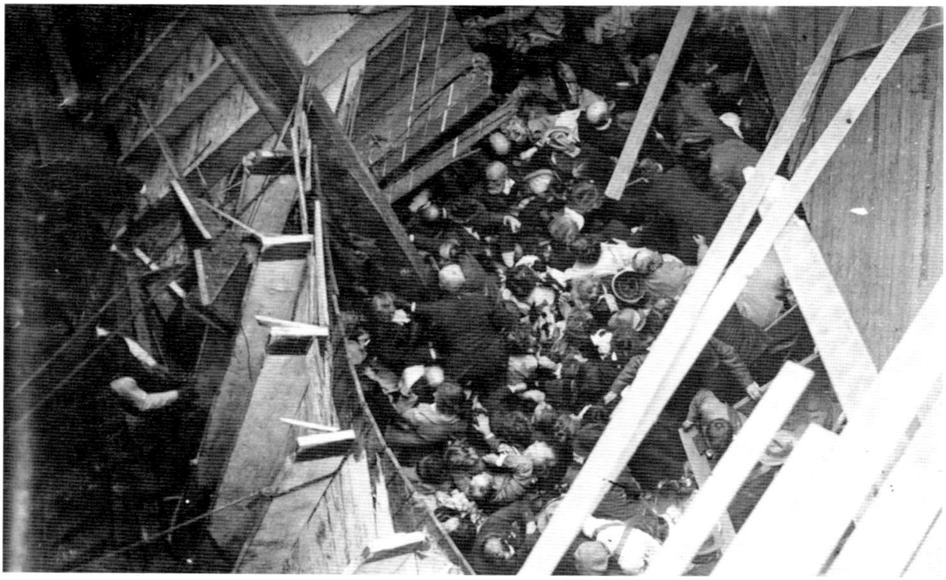

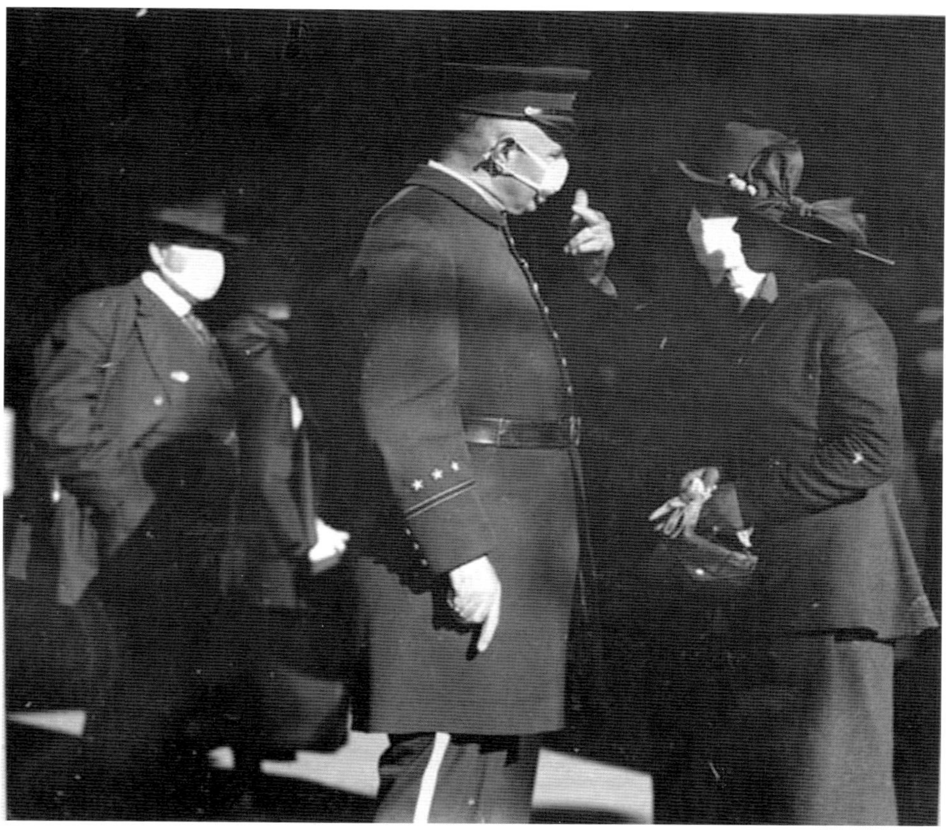

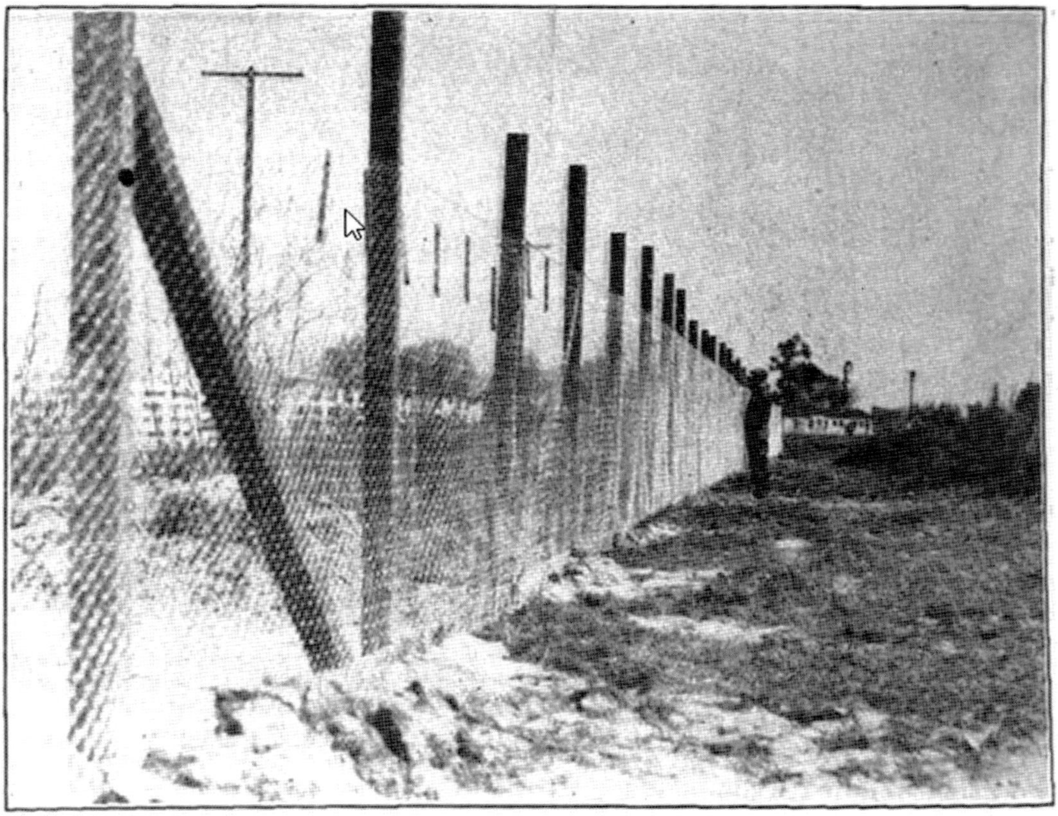

FIGURE 4.—Seven-foot chicken-wire fence around infected premises. A 24-hour guard system was maintained on all quarantined premises

Above: In 1929, Southern California was impacted by an outbreak of "hoof and mouth disease" among cattle, hogs and other livestock. FMD is one of the most contagious, infectious viral diseases of animals. Quarantine fences were placed in several places in Long Beach with guards stationed to keep people away from infected areas. (*USDA*)

Opposite above: The collapse of the Pine Avenue pier floors sent dozens to their deaths or serious injury during the 1913 "Empire Day" celebrations. A total of fifty were killed and 200 or more injured—mostly women. Makeshift tents were erected for a hospital and morgue. Some were taken to Long Beach Hospital and others to Seaside Hospital. (*LOC*)

Opposite below: Long Beach's public health officer, Dr. Ralph Taylor, worked with the City Council to impose restrictions on places where people would gather: churches, schools, theaters, moving picture shows, parks and the Pike. Local cemeteries have large sections dedicated to the babies and children who died from the flu. The federal government estimated that 1 million dollars a week was lost because of the closure of businesses. Police were utilized to enforce the wearing of surgical masks when people were in public as shown in the Library of Congress photograph.

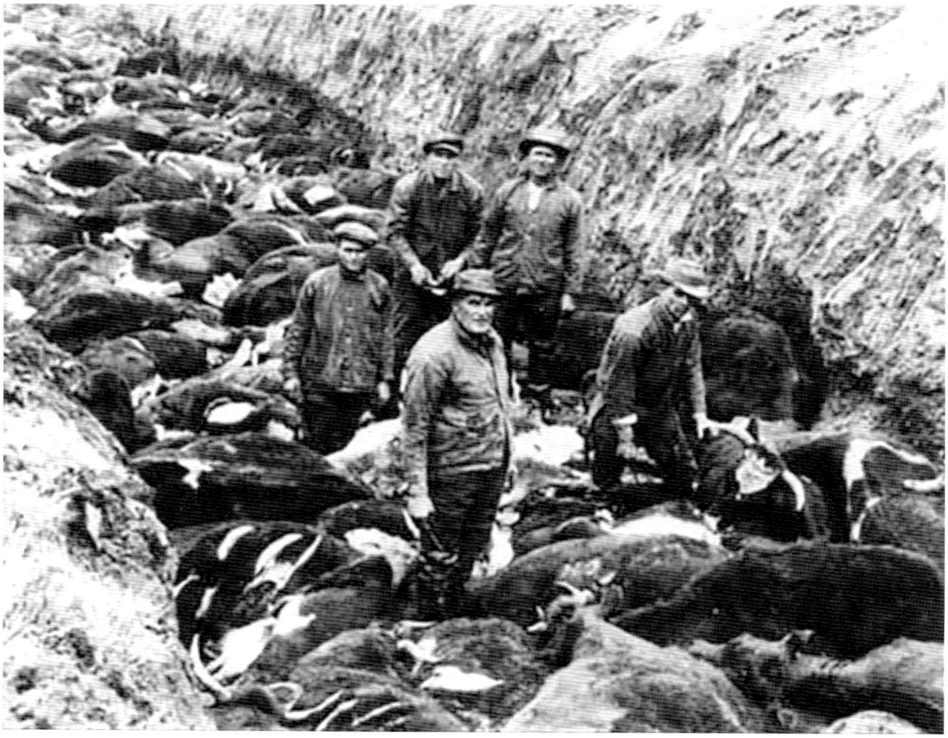

Above: When FMD struck, the Japanese hog farmers on Signal Hill had to kill their stock. Long Beach cattle owner, Llewellyn Bixby, ordered his men to dig deep trenches. His cows were pushed into the trenches and shot. In 1988, the land covering the trenches in east Long Beach began sinking under houses. Large bones were discovered when workers dug into the soil. (*USDA*)

Opposite above: The March 10, 1933, "Long Beach earthquake" caused massive destruction of brick houses, schools and other buildings. Seaside Hospital and St. Mary's Hospital sustained significant damage that would take several years to repair. (*USGS*)

Opposite below: The Long Beach Public Health Department has been in a variety of buildings. In early days, the public health officer worked out of his home or an office in City Hall. In the 1940s, it was located at 218 E. First Street (pictured) and then re-located in the 1950s to 2655 Pine Avenue, adjacent to Pacific Hospital. Today, the health department is at 2525 Grand Avenue. (*LBPL*)

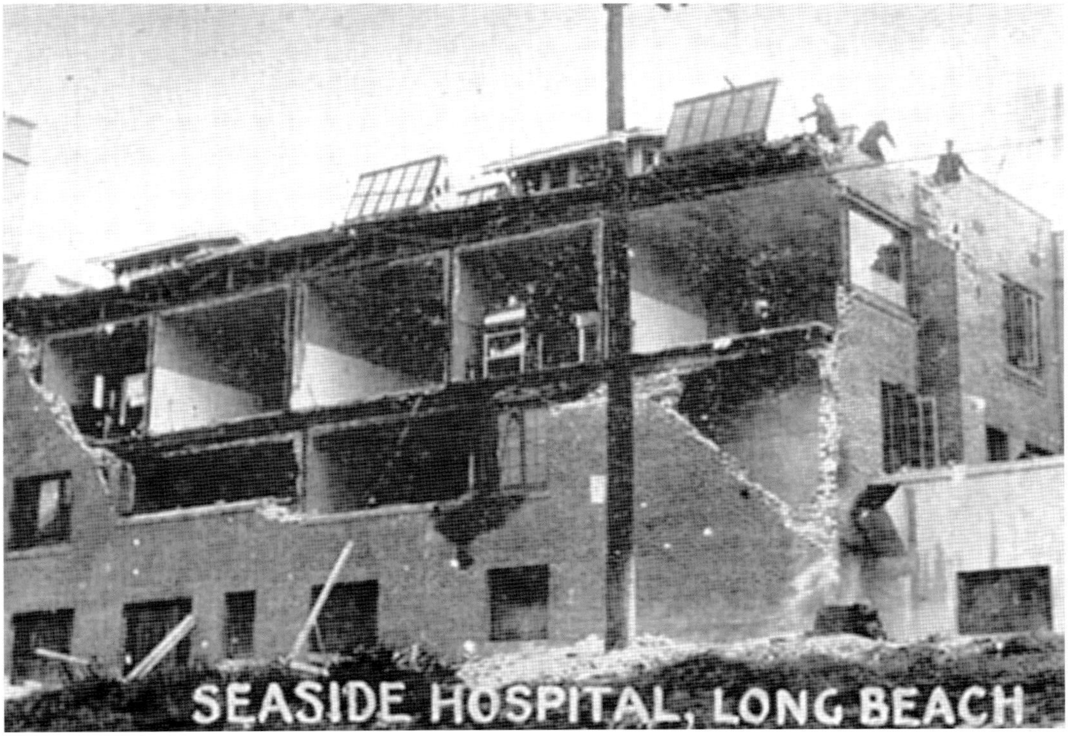
SEASIDE HOSPITAL, LONG BEACH

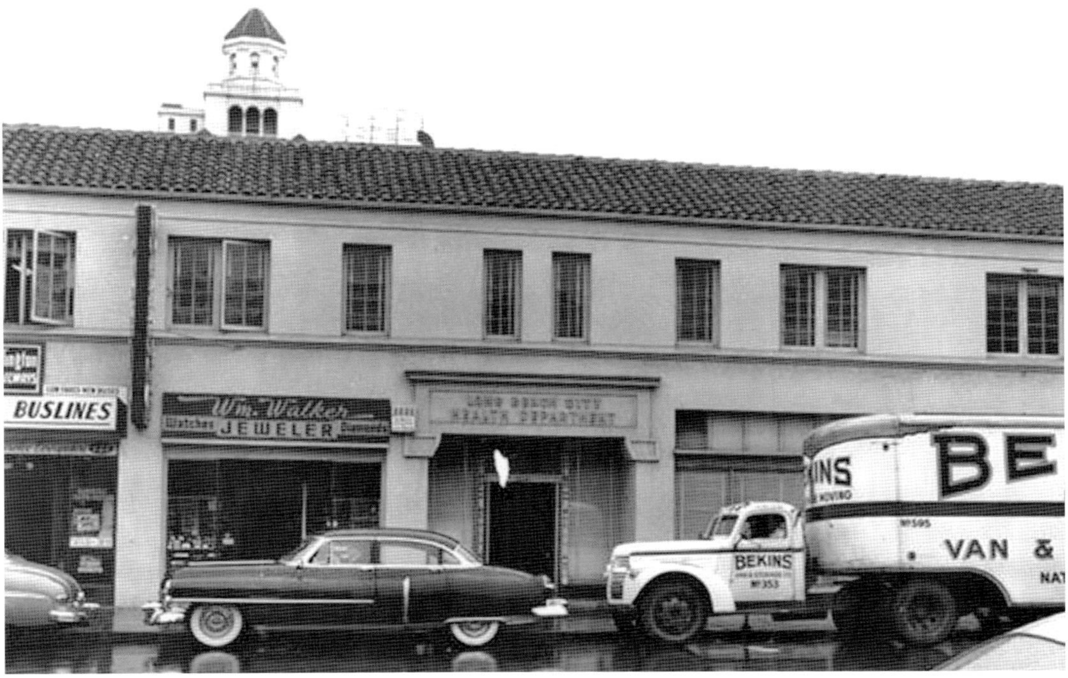
BUSLINES
Wm. Walker
Watches JEWELER Diamonds
LONG BEACH CITY
HEALTH DEPARTMENT
BEKINS
VAN &

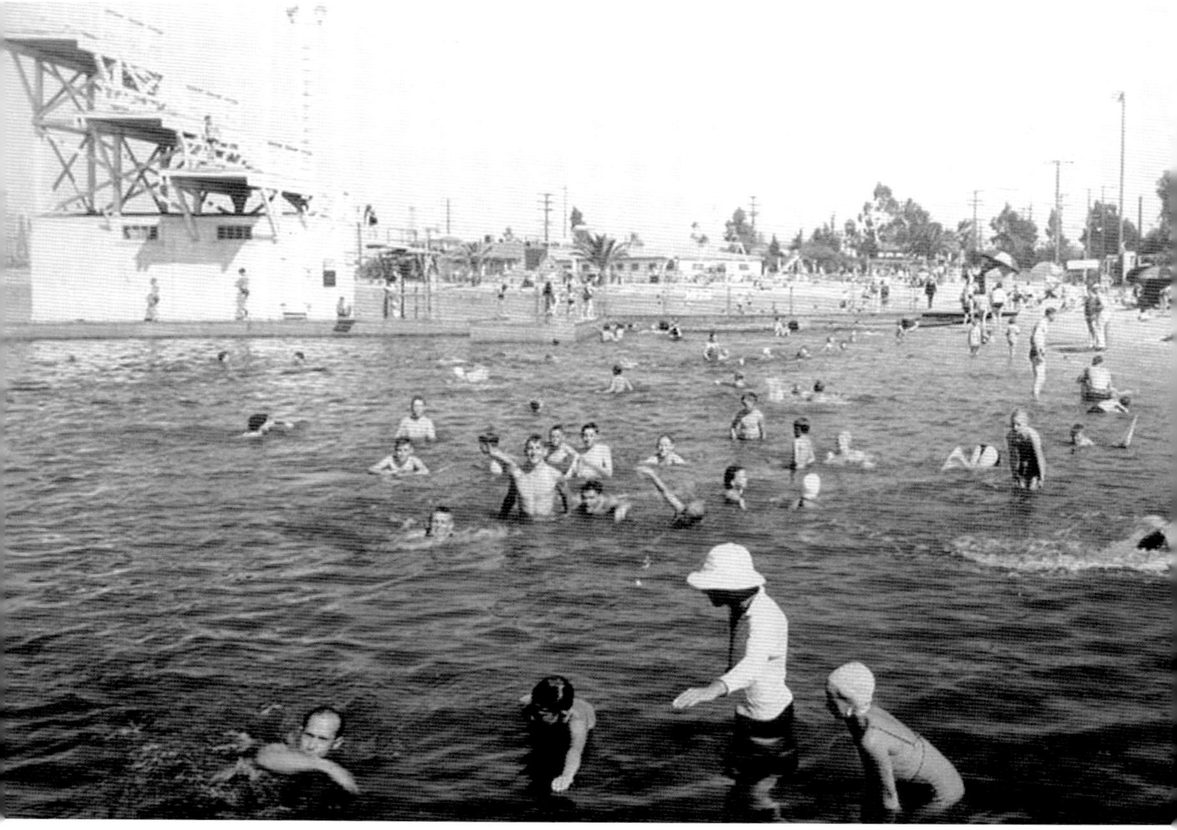

During the polio epidemic of the 1950s, parents kept their children away from public swimming pools and the Colorado Lagoon near Alamitos Bay. Because the saltwater lagoon did not have access to a free flow of water, it often became blocked with trash and other debris, resulting in stinky, murky water and was referred to as "polio pit." (*LBPL*)

Opposite: Illustration: *Notable Patients*

NOTABLE PATIENTS

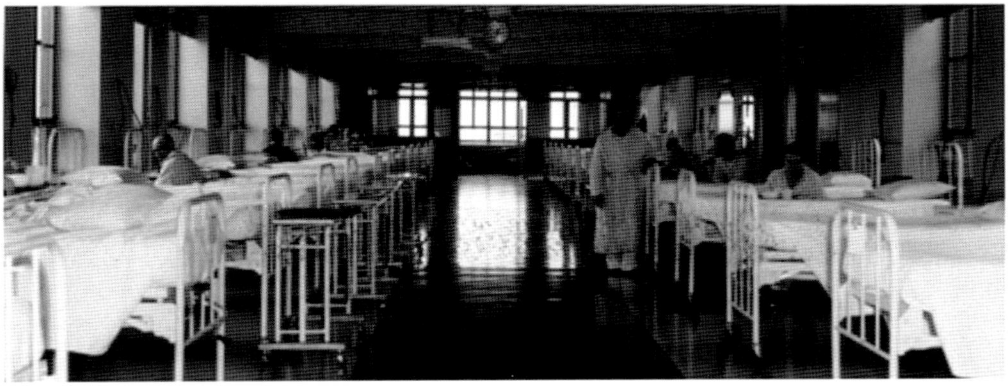

SEASIDE/MEMORIAL

- 1913 -- Mrs. A.E. Smith, Superintendent of Seaside, treated for injuries suffered in pier collapse
- 1916 -- Fire Chief J.E. Shrewsbury, died of injuries from automobile accident while responding to alarm
- 1920 -- Four workmen crushed when dome fell at the First Christian Church
- 1921 -- William Jennings Bryan Jr., treated for injuries caused by an automobile gas tank exploding
- 1924 -- Two women admitted in critical condition due to botched abortions
- 1930 -- Flossie Lewis gives birth to future Mayor of Long Beach, Beverly Lewis O'Neill
- 1936 -- Twenty-five treated after busses collide at Pine and 20th
- 1937 -- First quintuplets born in Long Beach
- 1954 -- Novelist James Hilton treated for terminal cancer
- 1974 -- Former Pres. Richard Nixon treated for exhaustion 45 days after his resignation

ST. MARY

- 1953 -- Former Governor Frank Merriam treated for automobile crash injuries
- 1957 -- Five workers treated for injuries suffered in tanker blast
- 1976 -- Four swimmers treated when roof of LB YWCA collapses on them

COMMUNITY

- 1930 -- Lt. Joseph Parents dies of injuries received when his Navy plane crashed into hangar at LB Airport
- 1939 -- Hospital founder and former Mayor of Long Beach, Fillmore Condit dies of "infirmities"
- 1952 -- Rancher and member of Long Beach pioneer family, Fred Bixby, is treated for heart ailment
- 1954 -- Edward Ledbetter, lone survivor of crash of Marine Corps jet that killed seven and destroyed four homes, dies

U.S. NAVAL

- 1945 -- Freed POW Navy Nurses, Lts. Ellen Page, Dorthy Still and Edwina Todd treated
- 1978 -- First Lady Betty Ford in alcohol and drug rehab

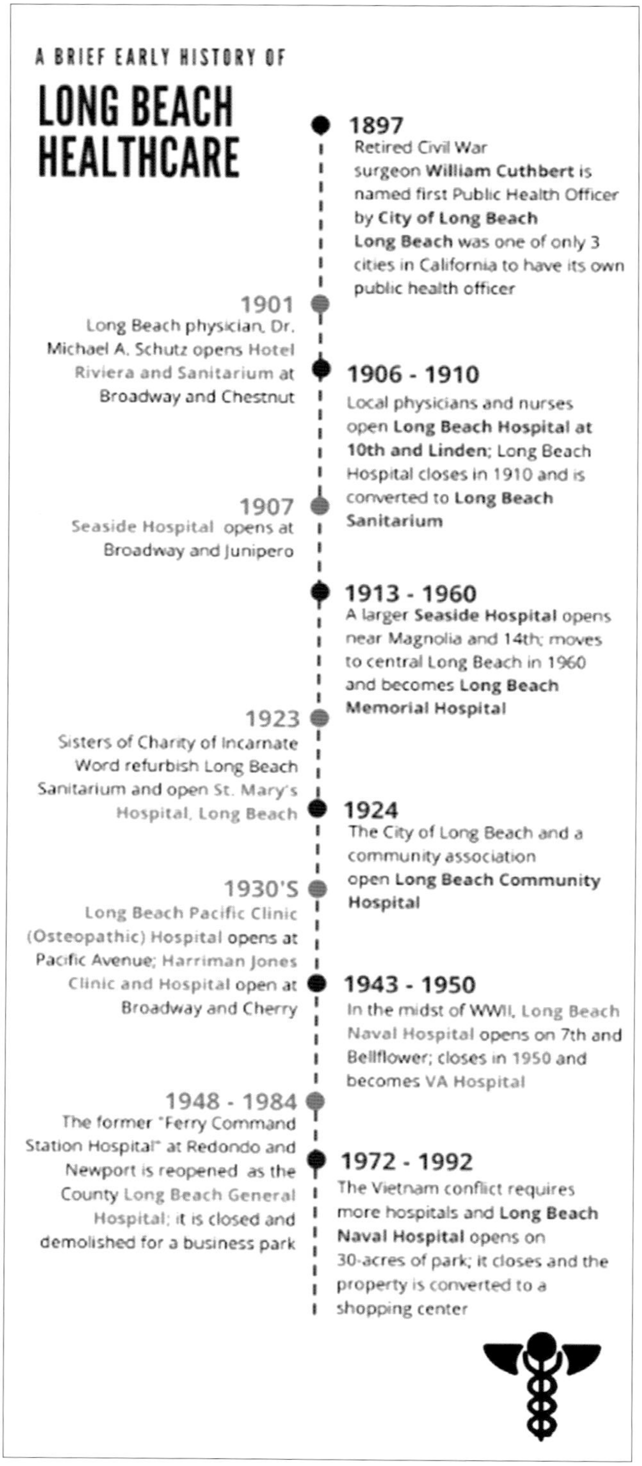

Illustration: *A Brief Early History of Long Beach Healthcare*

Bibliography

Photographs included were obtained from: Long Beach Public Library (LBPL); Los Angeles Public Library (LAPL); Library of Congress (LOC); California Library (CL); Historic Fresno (HF); US Geological Service (USGS); Memorial Care (MC); St. Anthony's Church History (SA); St. Mary Medical Center History (SMMC); US Patent Office (USPO); University of Southern California Archives (USC); Community Hospital of Long Beach Foundation Archives (CHLBF); Historical Society of Long Beach (HSLB); US Naval Archives (USNA); US Department of Agriculture (USDA), Others are from the author's personal collection or single collection.

Community Hospital of Long Beach History: https://www.chlbfoundation.org/history

Draft Environmental Impact Statement for the Disposal and Reuse of Naval Hospital in Long Beach, California, U.S. Navy, 1995

Condit, Fillmore, *My Wife and I*, self-published, 1921

Condit, Fillmore, *Activities*, self-published, 1932

Condit, Fillmore, *Prohibition and Health*, American Publishing Company, 1920

Historic Landmarks of Long Beach: https://goo.gl/ZkmZED

Decommissioning Ceremony of the U.S. Naval Hospital in Long Beach, California: https://goo.gl/tWzSqa

Holland, Mary Gardner, *Our Army Nurses: Stories from Women in the Civil War*, Minnesota: Edinborough Press, 1998

Jurman, Claudia and McCawley, William, *O, My Ancestor: Recognition and Renewal for the Gabrielino Tongva People of the Los Angeles Area*, Berkeley: Heyday Books, 2009

Indians of Southern California – Coastal Region: https://www.cabrillo.edu/~crsmith/anth6_scoastal_relig.html

Lane, M.A., *Dr. A. T. Still, Founder of* Osteopathy, Chicago: Osteopathic Publishing Company, 1918

McCready, Linda A., and Harris, Billie, *From Quackery to Quality Assurance: The First Twelve Decades of the MEDICAL BOARD OF CALIFORNIA*, California: Medical Board of California, 1995

Memorial Medical Center History, 50th Anniversary: https://goo.gl/Trmsv7

Schipske, Gerrie, *Early Long Beach*, South Carolina: Arcadia Publishing, 2011
Schipske, Gerrie, *Historic Cemeteries of Long Beach*, South Carolina: Arcadia Publishing, 2016
Schipske, Gerrie, *Early Aviation in Long Beach*, South Carolina: Arcadia Publishing, 2009
Sefinger, D.O., Michael, *The Merger: D.O.s and M.D.s in California*, www.xlibris.com, 2009
Forbes, DO, Henry, *Osteopathy's Legal Status Forever Established in California*, *Journal of Osteopathic Physician*, Volume XLI, January 1922, p. 4
St. Mary Medical Center History: *90-years-of-healing*: https://goo.gl/k6JEzp
Woolsey, Jane Stuart, *Reminiscence of a Civil War Nurse*, Minnesota: Edinborough Press